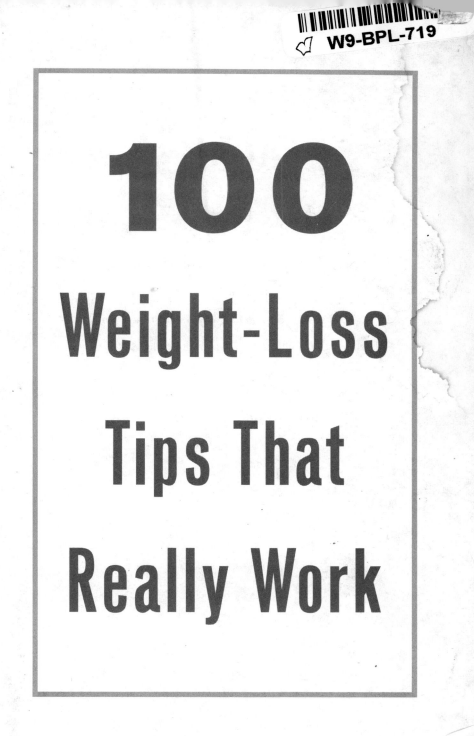

100
Weight-Loss
Tips That
Really Work

Also by Fred A. Stutman, M.D.

The Doctor's Walking Book

DIETWALK®: The Doctor's Fast 3-Day Superdiet

Walk, Don't Die

Walk to Win: The Easy 4-Day Diet and Fitness Plan

Diet-Step: 20 Grams/20 Minutes for Women Only!

Power Diet-Step:
Dr. Stutman's 14-Day Power Weight Loss & Fitness Plan

Diet Step: 30 Grams/30 Minutes for Seniors Only!

100 Best Fitness Tips

100
Weight-Loss Tips That Really Work

FRED A. STUTMAN, M.D.

New York Chicago San Francisco Lisbon London Madrid Mexico City
Milan New Delhi San Juan Seoul Singapore Sydney Toronto

The *McGraw-Hill* Companies

Library of Congress Cataloging-in-Publication Data

Stutman, Fred A.
     100 weight-loss tips that really work / Fred A. Stutman.
          p.   cm.
     Includes index.
     ISBN 0-07-147724-1 (alk. paper)
     1. Weight loss.   2. Reducing diets.   I. Title.   II. Title: One hundred
weight-loss tips that really work.

     RM222.2.S878   2007
     613.2'5—dc22   2006026547

DIET-STEP® is the registered trademark of Dr. Stutman's Weight-Loss and Fitness Program.
Reg. U.S. Pat. Off.
POWER DIET-STEP® is the registered trademark of Dr. Stutman's 21-Day Power Weight-Loss
and Fitness Plan.

     3 4 5 6 7 8 9 10 11 12 13 14 15 16 17 18 19   FGR/FGR   0 9 8 7

ISBN-13: 978-0-07-147724-6
ISBN-10:   0-07-147724-1

McGraw-Hill books are available at special quantity discounts to use as premiums and
sales promotions, or for use in corporate training programs. For more information, please
write to the Director of Special Sales, Professional Publishing, McGraw-Hill, Two Penn
Plaza, New York, NY 10121-2298. Or contact your local bookstore.

The information contained in this book is intended to provide helpful and informative
material on the subject addressed. It is not intended to serve as a replacement for
professional medical or fitness advice. Any use of the information in this book is at the
reader's discretion. The author and publisher specifically disclaim any and all liability
arising directly or indirectly from the use or application of any information contained in
this book. A health care professional should be consulted regarding your specific
situation.

This book is printed on acid-free paper.

To Suzanne,
Robert, Mary, Samantha, Alana,
Roni, Paul, Geoffrey,
Craig, Christine, Rain, India,
&
Sparkey

Contents

Part 3 ▪ Shed More Pounds with Protein

Part 4 ▪ Get the Skinny on Fat

Part 5 ▪ Power Foods to Put on Your Plate

Part 6 ▪ Diet Dos: Insider Secrets That Will Trim You Down

Part 7 ▪ Diet Don'ts: Don't Let These Diet Traps Trip You Up

Part 8 ▪ Try These Meals and Fat-Melting Tips in the Kitchen and On the Go

Part 9 ▪ Get Moving!

Introduction

I've been in practice for many years and have had an unending flow of patients looking for advice on how to successfully lose weight and keep it off. They invariably ask if the current fad diet is "The One" that will work, and they are always looking for that magic cure for being overweight and out of shape.

My response to their questions has been consistent over the years: "eat less and exercise more"! It's a simple formula, really, but dieters tend to look for something more extreme—the best-selling fad diet that is supposed to result in quick weight loss. I've researched many weight-loss programs and nutritional topics translating the science behind diet and nutrition into common sense easy-to-follow tips that I've broken out into the most common areas of concern.

100 Weight-Loss Tips That Really Work is a versatile book, a roadmap to success no matter how you pursue it. Read it from cover to cover for an overview on eating healthfully and exercising more. Or focus on those aspects of weight loss you struggle with or desire more information about. For extra motivation, try reading a tip a day and incorporating that advice into your daily menu or activity schedule.

Use the easy-to-prepare, good-tasting, and healthful meal and snack suggestions presented throughout the book to lose weight easily and maintain your ideal weight safely without the health dangers posed by unsafe low-carbohydrate and other fad diets. The emphasis is on walking as the best and most effective form of exercise, without the hazards of strenuous exercises. Busy people are offered numerous ways to fit walking into their daily routines. For example, parking at the far end of the lot and using the stairs instead of the elevator will burn additional fat calories. It all adds up to success for people who are too busy to diet or exercise.

Combined, the tips make for a doable set of building blocks for weight loss, physical fitness, and healthy eating habits. Choose the tips that are appropriate for your individual lifestyle.

The weight-loss tips in this book have been thoroughly researched for medical authenticity, are safe and effective, and provide you with a unique, easy-to-follow weight-loss system. You won't experience any rebound weight gain, and most important, you'll improve your health and add years to your life. You will feel better, look younger, have more energy, and lose weight with each and every weight-loss tip that you follow. The weight you lose will stay lost forever because you will have adopted more healthy eating and exercise habits that can last a lifetime.

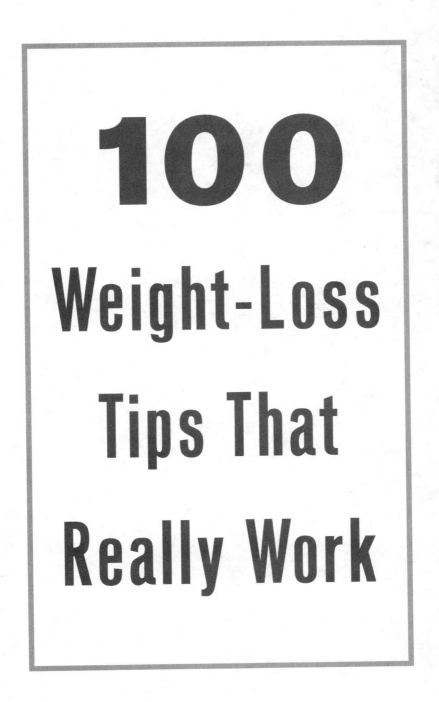

100

Weight-Loss

Tips That

Really Work

■

PART 1

Everything You Need to Know About Calories and Carbs

Tip 1 Calories Do Count

Despite what the latest fad diet says, there is a no magic formula to losing weight. You may be able to lose weight by following a variety of different diet programs; however, the only way to lose weight is to take in fewer calories than you burn. For permanent weight loss, eat healthful, nutritious foods and burn off extra calories with exercise.

A study published in the *Journal of American Medicine* in April 2003 found that consuming fewer calories on a daily basis over a long period of time is the most effective way to lose weight. A low-fat, high-fiber diet with moderate amounts of protein and complex carbohydrates is the single best healthy weight-loss diet that you can follow for good health and permanent weight loss. There are no dangerous side effects, no feelings of hunger, and along with permanent weight loss, you have the added health benefits of a balanced, nutritious diet.

In addition to losing weight, if you follow a low-fat, high-fiber diet you will have a lower incidence of heart disease, hypertension, strokes, and several forms of cancer. This diet, by its very nature, is a low-calorie diet in disguise, and what's more, it actually works and keeps on working. It is a diet plan that you can follow for a lifetime to lose weight, maintain your ideal weight, and enjoy good health, physical fitness, and longevity—one tip at a time!

Tip 2 Calculate Your Calorie Needs

There is an easy way to figure out how many calories you are eating every day to maintain your current weight. Multiply your current weight by 12, which will equal the number of calories needed daily to maintain your current weight. For example: if you weigh 150 pounds, multiply that by 12, which will equal 1,800 calories. 1,800 calories then is the number of calories you need every day to maintain your 150 pounds. If you weigh 125 pounds, multiply 125 × 12 = 1,500 calories, which means that a 125-pound person only needs 1,500 calories a day to maintain his or her 125-pound weight.

One easy technique for losing weight is to reduce your calorie intake by 300 calories per day and increase your activity level by 200 calories per day. This is a total of 500 calories lost per day. Since 3,500 calories equal one pound of fat, you will be able to lose one pound per week with little or no effort. That calculation is as follows: you are taking in 300 less calories per day and burning up 200 calories per day with activities such as walking, which equals 500 calories lost per day, × 7 days per week = 3,500 calories, which means you have lost one pound in one week. You can also reduce your calorie intake by 500 calories per day with no increase in your activity level and still lose a pound a week (500 calories reduced from diet × 7 days = 3,500 calories or one pound weight loss). Just think of the weight-loss possibilities there are if you decrease your calorie intake every day and increase your activity level!

Slow and steady weight loss from calorie adjustments is the safest and most effective way to lose weight and maintain that weight loss for life. This is because slow and steady weight loss conditions you to make permanent changes in your eating habits, and regular exercise conditions your body to expect regular physical activity every day for a feeling of well-being. Sound simple? It certainly is!

Tip 3   Try These Quick and Easy Ways to Cut Calories

Here are some helpful hints for you to cut calories without even noticing it!

- Drink one cup of fat-free milk instead of one cup of whole milk. Also try adding nonfat milk to your coffee, cappuccino, or lattes.
- Use one tablespoon of mustard, ketchup, or fat-free mayonnaise instead of regular mayonnaise in salads or on sandwiches.
- If you simply can't pass up the french fries or chips, try sharing a small serving with a friend, or just taste three or four and throw the rest away.
- Cut a slice of pizza in half and save the other half for later in the day.
- Pay careful attention to serving sizes of your favorite foods when you eat out. For example:
  - One-half cup of cooked cereal or pasta at home is equivalent to a single serving size; however, restaurant portions are equivalent to approximately three serving sizes—and that's before they even add the sauce to the pasta!
  - One-half of a bagel is one serving, but a deli bagel is equivalent to at least three servings. (A good way to cut calories and refined carbs is to scoop out the soft inside of the bagel, or a bread roll, before adding spread or sandwich ingredients.)

- One small pancake or waffle at home is equal to one serving size, but in a restaurant, one large pancake is about two and one-half servings.
- A dozen potato chips or tortilla chips equal approximately one serving; however, a small bag contains at least two to three servings.

- Always check the serving sizes on any prepackaged food you get. You may be surprised that some contain two or three servings. Most people assume that a package of processed foods is one serving size, when in actuality it may be two or three.
- Watch out for prepackaged foods that contain trans fats. They may not be listed or labeled on the package and are instead often identified as "partially hydrogenated" oils.
- When you order a meal in a restaurant, ask the waiter to wrap up half of the meal to go before you even start to eat. Don't wait until you've started the meal or you'll wind up unintentionally eating more than you meant to and your calorie count will go sky-high.
- Substitute low-fat, nonfat, or part-skim cheeses for the full-fat version. Low-fat goat cheese, feta, mozzarella, and ricotta cheese are good choices.
- Trim all visible skin and fat from poultry and meat before cooking.
- Avoid sugar in sodas, teas, and fruit drinks. Use fresh orange juice, grapefruit juice, tomato juice (low sodium), and non-caffeinated teas, coffee, and diet sodas for snack drinks. Or better yet, make water your drink of choice.
- Eat your meals more slowly. Take smaller, less frequent bites and chew each mouthful for a longer period of time. Pause between parts of the meal. This will give your body time to register fullness before you take in unnecessary calories.

Tip 4   Avoid Bad Carbs

Your body converts all of the carbohydrates that you eat into sugar (glucose), which our body's cells use as fuel. When glucose molecules pass from the intestines into the bloodstream, the organ known as the pancreas produces insulin, signaling to the body's cells to absorb the glucose. Once the cells (skin, internal organs, tissues, muscles, fat, and others) absorb the glucose, the insulin levels in the blood return to normal.

The main element that differentiates bad carbs from good carbs is how fast the carbohydrate foods are converted into sugar in the intestine and absorbed into the bloodstream. This is known as the *glycemic index*. Foods with a high glycemic index are considered to be the bad carbs. They include white flour and white rice, refined, highly processed flour (in white breads, cereals, spaghetti, macaroni, bagels, muffins, croissants, pastries, pretzels, pancakes, waffles); fruit juices, sugar-laden sodas, and sports drinks; cakes, pies, ice cream, cookies, candy, and most nonfruit desserts; chips and crackers; some vegetables (corn and white potatoes); sorbets, and sherbets.

Bad carbs are rapidly converted into glucose in the intestine, and then rapidly absorbed into the bloodstream. This rapid increase in blood sugar causes a rapid increase in insulin levels. Due to the output of insulin, blood glucose levels then rapidly decrease, actually starving the body's tissues and brain of energy. In response, the brain sends out hunger signals for another quick-fix meal to replenish the glucose in the blood. This vicious cycle leads to excessive calorie consumption, which invariably leads to excessive weight gain.

The increased insulin levels that are needed to fill the muscle and fat cells with sugar also inhibit the production of a muscle protein called *glucagon*. Glucagon signals the body's fat cells to burn stored fuel when the blood glucose levels fall below a critical level, causing the fat cells to store more fat instead of burning fat for the production of energy. Result: less energy produced, more fat stored.

In addition to gaining unwanted pounds, eating too many foods with a high glycemic index can cause serious health problems. When excess insulin is repeatedly produced by the pancreas in response to the ingestion of high-glycemic foods, the pancreas's insulin-producing cells can actually wear out, and then they begin to produce less and less insulin. This can eventually lead to diabetes and insulin resistance, a condition wherein the body's tissues resist insulin's signal to transfer glucose from the blood into the cells.

■ High-Sugar Diets May Increase the Risk of Breast Cancer

According to recent research reported in *The Journal of Cancer Epidemiology, Biomarkers & Prevention* (August 2004), women who eat a lot of refined carbohydrates have twice the risk of developing breast cancer of those women who eat less sugars and starches. Scientists think that an excess of refined carbohydrates in the diet may increase breast cancer risk by causing the blood sugar to rise rapidly, which in turn causes a surge in blood insulin levels. These high blood insulin levels can cause normal cells to divide too quickly and may cause higher levels of insulin in the breasts' cells. These two factors could possibly lead to the formation of cancer cells in the breast.

These studies don't suggest that people should go on the typical low-carbohydrate diet, but they do indicate that people should restrict refined carbohydrates and substitute complex high-fiber carbohydrates in their diets. High-fiber diets have been shown in many studies to decrease the risk of various types of cancer when combined with a low-fat lean protein diet. (High-fat diets, on the other hand, have been repeatedly shown to increase the risk of various forms of cancer, particularly breast cancer.) These findings raise concerns about women who eat excess amounts of refined sugars and could be at risk for developing breast cancer. This is particularly true for women who are overweight or diabetic or who have insulin resistance.

Tip 5 Count Calories, Not Carbs

We know there's no magic trick to losing weight; the only way to shed pounds is to take in fewer calories than you burn. The "trick" then, is to fuel your body without feeling deprived while reducing your calorie intake.

The body needs carbohydrates to function properly; what it doesn't need are excess calories in the form of refined sugars, starches, and saturated fats. The National Academy of Science Institute of Medicine's 2002 report on healthy eating (*Dietary Reference Intakes for Energy, Carbohydrate, Fiber, Fat, Fatty Acids, Cholesterol, Protein, and Amino Acids*) recommended that adults consume 45 to 65 percent of their calories from carbohydrates. This amounts to approximately 520 calories of carbohydrate daily, based on a 1,200 calorie diet.

Your body actually needs complex carbohydrates such as whole grains, fruits, and vegetables to function properly. These complex carbs are packed with nutrients and have far fewer calories than refined grains and sugar foods. Carbohydrates are broken down into glucose, a simple sugar that is the body and brain's preferred source of fuel. If you severely restrict carbohydrates as in low-carb diets, the stored carbohydrates in your muscles and liver get depleted also, and your body has to make glucose out of protein, which is an inefficient way to produce energy. This can lead to fatigue, depression, mineral imbalances, and protein loss from your body. Plus, these imbalances put a strain on the kidneys, liver, and other internal organs and can cause damage to organs if this type of diet is left unchecked.

Nutritionally empty carbs such as cookies, pastries, cakes, and ice cream are not only packed with sugar, but also contain considerable amounts of fat. For each gram of fat you consume, you are piling up 9 calories, compared with only 4 calories contained in a gram of carbohydrate or a gram of protein. So if you limit refined sugars, starches, and fatty foods, you will naturally cut calories from your diet and lose weight in a healthy fashion.

Tip 6 Concentrate on Complex Carbs

Carbohydrates have been getting a lot of bad press lately. Low-carb, Atkins-type diets lead many dieters to limit their carb intake or cut carbohydrates out altogether. Truth is, it's a better idea to concentrate on getting plenty of good, complex carbs in your diet. Here's why:

When you eat a low-carb, high-fat diet, all of the excess fat calories you eat are stored in fat cells and end up staying there indefinitely. The more fat you eat, the more fat your body retains. This occurs no matter how much you restrict your carbs; in fact, the more you limit your carb intake, the more fat you will consume. Low-carb diets are filled with fat, fat, and more fat—fat that not only fattens your face, abdomen, thighs, and buttocks, but also clogs your arteries with cholesterol. For more information on the low-carb trend, check out Tips 68 through 71.

On the other hand, by concentrating on eating good, complex carbs, you will lose weight safely and steadily and keep it off for good! Your body expends two and a half times more energy converting complex carbohydrates with a low glycemic index into your bloodstream for immediate use, and then into glycogen storage in your muscles and liver, than it expends converting fat into a source of fuel for energy production. In other words, a high complex carbohydrate, low-fat diet causes your body to work harder after each meal burning calories for energy than does a high-fat, low-carbohydrate diet. This results in a higher basal metabolic rate, *so that you burn an additional 250 calories daily* by the simple thermic effect of converting carbohydrates into energy—talk about a healthy and easy way to burn extra calories!

Tip 7 Lose Weight with Good Carbs

According to a new Harvard study, women who eat at least two servings daily of high-fiber whole-grain breads and cereals are 50 percent less likely to gain weight compared to those who eat refined carbohydrates, or bad carbs, that lack fiber. High-fiber good carbs burn more calories during digestion and make you feel fuller earlier and longer than refined bad carbs. High-fiber breads, cereals, pastas, and rice all reduce the output of fat-storing insulin, which results in less weight gained and more fat calories burned.

Most vegetables (except corn and white potatoes), whole fruits, beans, legumes, nuts, and whole-grain cereals and breads have a low glycemic index and can be considered good carbs. As your body converts these good carbohydrates into glucose, they are slowly processed in the intestinal tract and absorbed into the bloodstream. Because this glucose is absorbed gradually, it only triggers a moderate, sustained rise in the insulin produced by the pancreas. This even level of blood insulin can process the glucose into the body's cells slowly for use in energy production. In other words, you avoid high levels of glucose that fill your cells with extra sugar, as well as the rapid fluctuation in blood glucose levels that cause excess hunger, carbohydrate cravings, and excessive weight gain.

So eating good carbs can actually help you lose weight, provided they are contained in low-fat, low-calorie foods. Plus, these good-carb foods are primarily of plant origin and contain fiber as well as many different phytonutrients, or nutrients from plant sources, including essential vitamins, minerals, and enzymes.

Tip 8   Try These Tasty, Good-for-You Carbs

The following carbohydrate foods all have a low glycemic index and make a tasty addition to a healthy diet:

- Vegetables are essential to a healthy diet. Most vegetables, with the exception of corn and white potatoes, are great sources of good carbs.
- Whole fruits are another great way to get good-tasting good carbs into your diet. Just be wary of fruits with high sugar contents such as watermelon and grapes, and fruit juices, which contain high levels of sugar and very little actual fruit.
- Beans and legumes are good carbs as well as excellent sources of fiber, protein, vitamins, minerals, and nutrients.
- Whole grains are another great source of good carbs. These include:
  - Whole-grain cereals such as oatmeal (but be careful—flavored instant oatmeal may have a high sugar content) or cold cereals. Make sure that the package shows a fiber content of at least 4 to 5 grams of fiber or more per serving and a sugar count lower than 10 to 12 grams of sugar per serving, preferably under 8 grams. Whole-grain cereals that contain bran are usually high in fiber.
  - Whole-grain breads, especially those that also contain bran. The label on whole-grain breads should show that the first ingredient listed is "whole-grain flour" (for example "whole wheat flour"). If it doesn't list whole-grain flour first, then it is really not a whole-grain bread.
  - Whole wheat pastas. These now come in many varieties, such as noodles, spaghetti, vermicelli, and linguini, so you can be creative with your healthy pasta dishes!

- Brown long-grain rice. Brown rice makes a good low-glycemic addition to any meal since it is broken down and absorbed slowly.
- Nuts. Nuts such as almonds, walnuts, cashews, pecans, and hazelnuts (see Tip 44) make great low-glycemic snack foods. In addition to being absorbed slowly, they are excellent sources of protein, fiber, magnesium, copper, folic acid, potassium, and vitamin D. Nuts also contain monounsaturated fats, "good fats" that help to keep blood vessels open and can reduce the risk of heart disease and strokes. Raw nuts are particularly heart-healthy because they contain generous amounts of omega-3 fatty acids. These omega-3 fatty acids are heart protective and also help prevent certain forms of cancer.

PART 2

■

Fiber Up to Trim Down

Tip 9 Not All Carbs Are Created Equal

Fiber, commonly known as bulk or roughage, is the part of plant foods that cannot be digested completely, so that it passes through the digestive tract intact. Fiber is not found in foods of animal origin such as meat or dairy products. Bacteria present in the colon are able to partly digest fiber through a process known as fermentation.

Types of Fiber

Plant foods contain a mixture of different types of fibers. These fibers can be divided into soluble or insoluble, depending on their solubility in water.

Insoluble Fiber

Insoluble fibers make up the structural parts of the cell walls of plants and come in three major types: cellulose, hemicelluloses, and lignin. These fibers absorb many times their own weight in water, creating a soft bulk to the stool and hastening the passage of waste products out of the body. Insoluble fibers promote bowel regularity and aid in the prevention and treatment of some forms of constipation, hemorrhoids, and diverticulitis. These fibers also may decrease the risk of colon cancer by diluting potentially harmful substances that are present in the colon.

Soluble Fiber

Soluble fibers are easily digested and come in three major types: gums, pectins, and mucilages. Soluble fibers are found within the plant cells. When ingested, these fibers form a gel that slows the speed at which the stomach empties and the speed at which simple sugars are absorbed from the intestine. This process helps to regulate blood sugar levels, which is particularly helpful for people with diabetes and is helpful in controlling weight for both diabetics and nondiabetics.

When your stomach empties more slowly, you feel fuller, experience a decrease in hunger, and ultimately consume fewer calories. For example, if you eat a high-fiber apple, you'll feel fuller than you will if you eat a fiberless cupcake, despite the fact that they are approximately the same weight and size and the cupcake contains many more calories. In fact, it would take approximately *three* cupcakes to satisfy your brain's hunger center before you realized that you were full—and by then you would already have consumed 480 calories and 16.5 grams of fat.

Many soluble fibers can also assist in lowering blood cholesterol by binding with bile acids and cholesterol and eliminating the cholesterol through the intestinal tract before it can be absorbed into the bloodstream. The best sources of soluble fiber are fruits and vegetables, oat bran, barley, dried peas and beans, flaxseed, and psyllium.

The Function of Fiber

The most important function of dietary fiber is to bind water in the intestine, in the form of a gel. This gel prevents the overabsorption of water from the large intestine and ensures that the stool content of the large bowel is both bulky and soft, and consequently, its passage through the intestine is not delayed. Another important function of fiber is its effect on the metabolism, absorption, and reabsorption of bile acids and cholesterol. Dietary fiber binds or attaches to both cholesterol and bile acids and consequently decreases their absorption from the bowel. It is now recognized that a number of diseases are, at least in part, caused by a lack of dietary fiber, including gastrointestinal, metabolic, cardiovascular, and degenerative disorders including some cancers and neurological diseases. This was first described in 1975 in P. D. Burkitt and H. C. Trowell's book *Refined Carbohydrate Foods and Disease* (New York/London: Academic Press).

There is almost an inverse relationship between the amount of fiber consumed and the prevalence of the various diseases in different countries. The higher the intake of dietary fiber, the lower the incidence of the above-named disorders.

■ **Health-Protecting Phytochemicals Found in High-Fiber Foods**

The latest medical reports on high-fiber foods indicate that some dark green and dark yellow vegetables and fruits contain cancer-protecting substances called phytonutrients. One substance, known as beta-carotene (a nutrient that the body converts into vitamin A), is found in high concentration in spinach, carrots, broccoli, brussels sprouts, cauliflower, winter squash, cabbage, oranges, grapefruit, apricots, and peaches. These high-fiber foods also contain large amounts of vitamin C. Both vitamins may be protective against cancer of the lung, esophagus, stomach, large bowel, and skin.

How Fiber Helps You Lose Weight

Fiber has the amazing ability to prevent some of the fat you eat from being stored as fat in your body. When you combine high-fiber foods with any fat in your diet, like a piece of cake or a hamburger, each gram of fiber traps some of the fat by entwining it in a web made up of thousands of fiber strands. Once the fat is trapped in the fiber's web, it passes through the intestinal tract before it is absorbed into the bloodstream. Fiber actually removes fat from your body the way a garbage truck removes garbage!

In addition, high-fiber foods have a high bulk ratio, which satisfies the hunger center more quickly than low-fiber foods; consequently, fewer calories are consumed. Fiber-rich foods take longer to chew and to digest than fiber-depleted foods, which gives your stomach time to feel full. Feeling full earlier leads to consuming fewer calories. High-fiber foods also contain fewer calories for their volume. Fiber-rich foods such as fruits and vegetables, whole-grain cereals and breads, yams and sweet potatoes, and legumes are low in fat calories and have a high water content. You are, therefore, eating less and enjoying it more.

Tip 10 Burn More Calories with Fiber

Who says dieting has to be hard work? We know that dietary fiber helps you lose weight by blocking the absorption of fat in your body. In addition to helping flush fat through your body, dietary fiber will actually help you burn extra calories. It sounds too good to be true, but it really works!

Fiber burns up calories by itself. This is accomplished because your intestinal tract works harder to digest fiber foods. The body's metabolism therefore uses more energy for this time-consuming digestion, and as a result can burn most of the calories that the fiber foods contain. Strange as it seems, some heavily fibered foods can even burn up more calories than they contain, thereby creating a deficit of calories. This causes the body to use stored body fat for the production of energy.

Each gram of fiber you consume can burn up approximately 9 calories, most of which come from fat. So if you eat 30 grams of fiber a day, you can burn up an additional 270 calories daily (30 grams fiber × 9 calories). You can subtract those 270 calories every day from your total daily calorie intake, without actually cutting those calories from your diet in order to lose weight.

In addition to blocking fat and burning calories, fiber foods bind with water in the intestinal tract and form bulk that makes you feel full early in the course of your meal. So you eat less, and therefore you consume fewer calories at each meal. Also, your appestat, or hunger mechanism, is satisfied for longer periods of time, since it takes longer to digest fiber foods, and therefore you will have less of a tendency to snack between meals.

Tip 11 Avoid Refined Grains and Other Low-Fiber Foods

Eating excessive amounts of low-fiber foods will invariably cause weight gain. Fiber-deficient foods such as fats, refined sugars, flour, and alcohol require minimal chewing, have little or no bulk content, and are, in most cases, considerably more concentrated in calories than high-fiber foods. Low-fiber foods enter the intestinal tract more rapidly, where they are quickly absorbed as sugars. This rapid rise in blood sugar causes a spike in insulin production, which stores more fat in the body and then quickly drops the blood sugar, which in turn makes you hungry again. Because these low-fiber foods have no bulk and a higher calorie concentration, you have to consume large amounts of these foods—and large amounts of calories—before your hunger is satisfied.

A high-fiber diet is essentially a healthy, low-fat diet, which decreases the intake of refined and processed food. This encourages the consumption of fresh fruits, vegetables, and whole-grain cereals and breads.

Have the Orange Instead of the Orange Juice

Removing the healthy fiber from food, such as refining grains or flours to make white bread, white rice, pasta, and cereal, or extracting the juices out of whole fruits and vegetables, results in the following negative features:

- Healthy high-fiber foods become less healthy low-fiber foods.
- Low-calorie foods become high-calorie foods.

- High-bulk foods turn into low-bulk foods.
- Longer eating time changes into shorter eating time, making it easy to consume too many calories.
- Hunger-satisfying foods lose their ability to easily satisfy hunger.
- Good, complex carbs that are slowly absorbed into the bloodstream become simple sugars that are quickly absorbed, resulting in increased insulin production and subsequent weight gain.

Dietary fiber takes longer to chew and eat, fills you up, and satisfies your hunger without excessive calorie consumption. High-fiber diets may also reduce the amount of calories absorbed from the food that is eaten. High-fiber diets are often referred to as having a low energy density and will help prevent excessive caloric intake. Take advantage of these benefits by choosing high-fiber complex carbohydrates rather than low-fiber processed alternatives.

Tip 12 Get Your Fiber 2 Grams at a Time

When you're trying to eat a high-fiber diet, it helps to have a general idea of which fruits, grains, and veggies will give you the most bang for your buck. So here's a list of high-fiber foods with their fiber content.

Fiber-Filled Fruits

Each serving of these fruits has approximately 2 grams of fiber:

1 apple or pear	1½-ounce box raisins
1 banana	1 medium peach
½ cup strawberries	2 small plums
1 small orange	10 large cherries

2 Grams a Grain

Each serving of these breads has approximately 2 grams of fiber:

Whole wheat bread	Bran muffin (low fat)
Cracked wheat bread	Stone-ground whole wheat bread

Chock-Full-of-Fiber Cereals

Each serving of these healthful cereals has approximately 2 grams of fiber:

½ biscuit shredded wheat	½ cup oatmeal
1⅓ cups puffed wheat	½ cup wheat bran
⅔ cup cornflakes	½ cup Grape Nuts

Cereals that are really high in fiber include 40% Bran, All-Bran, Grape Nuts, Fiber One, Shredded Wheat, Whole Wheat Flakes, Raisin Bran, Multigrain Cheerios, and Multigrain Chex. Check the ingredients label and look for 5 or more grams of dietary fiber on the label.

Very Good-for-You Veggies

Each serving of these vegetables has approximately 2 grams of fiber:

1 cup celery	2 cups lettuce
1 ear corn on the cob	½ cup green beans
½ cup baked beans	1 medium potato
1 medium raw tomato	4 brussels sprouts
1 stalk broccoli	⅓ cup carrots

Of all vegetables, artichokes, green beans, cabbage, cauliflower, brussels sprouts, dried beans, lima beans, and peas are the highest in fiber.

Spreads and Sides

Each serving of these favorite spreads and sides has approximately 1 gram of fiber.

2½ teaspoons peanut butter	10 peanuts
1 tablespoon strawberry jam	1 large pickle
1 cup popcorn	2 teaspoons relish

Tip 13   Start Your Day with a Bowl of Heart-Healthy, High-Fiber Cereal

New findings show that fiber, especially the fiber in cereal products, protects against heart disease. In *The Nurses' Health Study*, which examined the fiber consumption of seventy thousand women from 1984 to 1998, the women who ate an average of 23 grams of fiber a day had a 47 percent lower risk of major coronary events, including myocardial infarction and/or fatal coronary heart disease, compared to those who ate about half as much fiber. A daily bowl of cold whole-grain breakfast cereal that supplies 5 or more grams of fiber cut heart disease risk by approximately 37 percent (*JAMA* 282, no. 16; October 27, 1999).

When researchers analyzed the individual effects of three different fiber sources (fruits, vegetables, and cereals), it was found that cereal fiber, more than any other type of fiber, significantly reduced the risk of heart disease. Whole-grain products may increase the body's sensitivity to insulin and thus lower the triglyceride levels. Whole-grain products, especially soy-based cereals, are an important source of phytoestrogens and may favorably affect blood coagulation activity.

In a recent article in the *Archives of Internal Medicine* (164: 370–376; 2004), it was reported that fruit and cereal fiber might decrease the risk of heart disease. The authors thought that the fiber contained in fruit and cereals can lower blood cholesterol and blood pressure, improve insulin sensitivity, and also make the blood less likely to clot.

Vegetable fiber, however, did not show the same reduced risk of coronary heart disease, which may have been attributed to the failure to distinguish between starchy vegetables (corn and potatoes) and nonstarchy vegetables (broccoli and cauliflower). However, due to its high plant nutrient content, vegetable fiber is still extremely important in the reduction of a whole host of degenerative diseases.

This particular study pooled data from ten other studies in the United States and Europe that included almost 100,000 men and 250,000 women. The purpose of the study, supported by the National Health, Lung and Blood Institute and the Danish Medical Council, was to determine if dietary fiber actually caused a significant decrease in heart disease. Over an eight-year follow-up, the risk of coronary heart disease was 10 to 30 percent lower for each 10 grams of total fruit or cereal fiber consumed daily. Cereal and fruit for breakfast is truly a heart-healthy meal.

Fiber-rich oatmeal or a cold bran cereal with skim or 1 percent milk is a great way to start your morning diet. These cereals are nutritious, taste great, and are slow to digest. The high insoluble fiber content of whole-grain cereals causes your appetite mechanism to shut down early because of its slow rate of absorption from the intestinal tract. These good-tasting whole-grain cereal products have also been shown to reduce cravings for high refined sugar products and fatty foods such as midmorning doughnut or coffee cake snacks.

Oatmeal in particular is also high in soluble fiber, which helps to clean out the fat from your blood vessels by increasing the HDL cholesterol, which sweeps the bad LDL cholesterol from the bloodstream. Oatmeal for breakfast has been recommended by the American Heart Association as a great start for your day to reduce your risk of heart disease while it reduces your waistline. People who eat oatmeal or other whole-grain bran cereals daily have less than one-half the risk of developing obesity and diabetes as those who don't. High-fiber bran cereals help to regulate insulin production in the morning, which helps control your appetite and reduce the risk of gaining unwanted pounds.

Bran cereals are also packed with magnesium, which is a mineral that can also reduce your risk of developing diabetes. Magnesium also helps to stabilize your blood sugar by preventing the overproduction of insulin by the pancreas.

Fiber Knocks Out Heart Disease

In a recent study in the *American Journal of Clinical Nutrition*, women who ate three to four servings of whole grains a day had one-third to one-half the risk of developing heart disease compared to women who ate refined flour, such as white bread. It is important to check the ingredients in any commercial food to see that it is truly made from whole grains. In particular, it is important to check the ingredients in snack foods like cookies, crackers, and chips, since many of these products contain not only refined white flour, but also partially hydrogenated oils (trans fats), which can raise your cholesterol more than any other type of saturated fats.

Tip 14 Enjoy These Appetite-Reducing Foods

Oranges and grapefruit contain soluble and insoluble fiber along with a form of fiber called pectin. The pectin fiber in these fruits suppresses your appetite and has only 70 calories. Oranges and grapefruit also contain many plant nutrients that help to lower blood fats and strengthen your immune system. (Eight ounces of orange or grapefruit juice, on the other hand, contain approximately 130 to 150 calories and are loaded with sugars, which cause your insulin levels to spike and results in sugar being metabolized into fat cells.)

Apples are another natural hunger suppressant, since they contain soluble and insoluble fiber, including pectin. One medium apple with the skin contains approximately 4 grams of fiber that combines with water in your digestive tract to form bulk in the intestines, which decreases your hunger and will make you feel full earlier and stay satisfied longer. At the same time, the pectin suppresses your appetite by tricking your brain's hunger center (appestat) into believing that you are full, when all you've really eaten is one delicious apple. This multifiber food fills you up without filling you out, and the high fiber content helps to lower your blood pressure, lower your blood cholesterol, and has been shown to decrease the incidence of colon polyps and colon cancer.

In contrast, eating a piece of cake, which has no fiber and lots of sugar, never stimulates the appestat to shut down, and consequently your body doesn't register fullness before you have had time to consume two or three pieces of cake. The same goes for cheeseburgers, french fries, and empty calories like soft drinks. This is because these foods contain lots of fat and/or refined carbohydrates, which are absorbed quickly and increase the blood sugar and blood insulin levels, which then leads to hunger.

Apple cider vinegar is another great appetite-reducer. It contains several acids called malic and tartaric acid that act as digestive enzymes and help to break down carbohydrates slowly, which in turn slows their absorption into the bloodstream. The tart flavor of apple cider vinegar also increases the production of saliva, which contains enzymes that aid in slower digestion of carbohydrates as well. Try adding one tablespoon of apple cider vinegar to salads for its appetite-suppressing effect. Nonfat raspberry vinaigrette dressing also contains some of these appetite-suppressing components. Any type of vinegar dressing, such as balsamic vinaigrette, has the ability to suppress your appetite. Just remember to use oil-based dressings sparingly, or else the calories from the oil will start to build up.

Tip 15 Try These Easy Ways to Sneak More Fiber into Your Diet

Fiber produces its most beneficial effect when it is eaten with each meal of the day. It is also important to drink six to eight glasses of water daily. Fiber can absorb many times its own weight of water, providing bulk to the diet and a subsequent feeling of fullness. Here are nine easy ways to fiber up your diet:

- Use whole-grain or fiber-enriched breads, which have more than double the fiber content of white bread. Some great options are cracked wheat bread, whole wheat pita, rye, and pumpernickel. Avoid high-fat, low-fiber breads such as French, Italian, and white bread, garlic bread, and rolls.
- Consume more salads (without high-fat dressing, of course; try using a little olive oil and vinegar). Include ingredients like tomatoes, carrots, celery, mushrooms, spinach, and the many varieties of lettuce.
- Add garden vegetables like cabbage, broccoli, brussels sprouts, green beans, onions, corn, and peas to your diet.
- Try legumes such as lentils, dried beans, and baked beans without added sugar or bacon.
- Try adding bran, nuts, seeds, or grits to soups, yogurt, or casseroles for an extra boost of fiber.
- Use whole-grain flour or soy flour instead of refined white flour whenever possible.
- Use whole-grain products like brown long-grain rice and whole-grain noodles.

- Eat more whole fruits like apples, oranges, pears, bananas, strawberries, blueberries, plums, peaches, and cherries.
- Sprinkle unprocessed bran and wheat germ on cereal or other foods, or mix them with orange or tomato juice. Each level teaspoon of dry bran or wheat germ powders contains 2 grams of dietary fiber, making them a convenient way to add fiber to foods.

Start slowly when adding fiber to your diet to avoid cramping, bloating, or gas. Make small additions of fiber-rich foods over a period of four to six weeks. If you find that a particular high-fiber food causes cramping or bloating, discontinue eating it and try another type of high-fiber food. Continue to increase your daily fiber intake until you reach between 25 and 30 grams of fiber a day for good health and weight reduction.

Remember, it's very important to drink more fluids—six to eight glass daily—as you increase your fiber intake. Fiber can absorb many times its own weight in water. This provides bulk to the diet, which makes you feel full so that you cut down on the total number of calories that you consume daily. This excess bulk formed by fiber and water also helps to keep your intestinal tract healthy.

Tip 16 Try These Fiber–Filled Snacks That Keep the Scale Happy

Fruits and vegetables; whole-grain crackers, breads, and cereals; soups with lots of vegetables; 100 percent vegetable juices; nuts and dried fruits; and popcorn are all high-fiber snacks that keep weight off and satisfy your appetite. These fiber-filled snacks take longer to digest, satisfying your appetite for a longer period of time

Stay away from snack foods that contain refined carbohydrates like cookies, pretzels, crackers, and candies. These refined sugars increase your appetite by spiking both blood sugar and insulin levels and help to store unwanted fat in your abdomen, buttocks, and thighs.

Next time you're in the mood for a snack, go for one that will fill you up without filling you out!

- Soups with lots of veggies make an excellent midday snack for appetite control; just steer clear of creamed soups that will have a higher fat content. Several companies have come out with new travel-type containers for soups that can be eaten on the go, with or without heating.
- One hundred percent vegetable juices come in plastic travel bottles and make an excellent high-fiber snack that's also chock-full of essential nutrients, vitamins, and minerals.
- Fruits and veggies make for an excellent high-fiber, nutritious, appetite-satisfying snack that you can take with you anywhere. Dried fruits such as figs, prunes, and apricots also are great travel snacks that are high in fiber, low in calories and fats, and high in essential nutrients, vitamins, and miner-

als. These fruit and veggie travel packs are loaded with nutrients such as B-complex vitamins, potassium, folic acid, magnesium, and iron, among others.

• For an energy punch, try a high-fiber/protein combo. As explained in Part 3, combining your high-fiber snack with lean protein will boost your energy and help keep weight off. Some delicious options are peanut butter with low-sugar jelly; low-fat cheese on whole wheat crackers, bread, or pita; and low-fat turkey or cheese on a slice of whole wheat bread or a whole-grain English muffin. Stay away from packaged snacks like peanut butter crackers, which are loaded with unhealthy trans fats.

• High-fiber cereal makes an excellent transportable, nutritious snack to take with you anywhere. Add some dried fruit for additional flavor and nutrition. Even the varieties of cereals that are lightly sweetened are great diet snacks provided they're high-fiber, whole-grain, low-sugar and low-fat cereals. Make sure the cereal has at least 5 grams or more of dietary fiber.

Tip 17 Eat These High-Fiber Foods That Pack a Nutritional Punch

Here are a few fiber-filled favorites to try that have many nutritional benefits as well as great taste:

- Spinach and dark green leafy vegetables are naturally low in calories and fill you up with their fiber content and their crunch factor. Plus because they take longer to eat your brain has time to register fullness before you've had time to load up on calories. Green leafy vegetables also contain many plant nutrients, antioxidants, and B-complex vitamins, which help to prevent cancer, heart disease, and degenerative neurological diseases.
- Tomatoes are unique in their ability to produce an amino acid called *carnitine*. This amino acid increases your body's basal metabolic rate, causing your body to burn fat at a faster rate. Any and all tomato products, from ketchup to tomato sauce, are great for your weight-reducing diet. Tomatoes also contain abundant amounts of vitamin C and an antioxidant called *lycopene*, which helps to prevent several types of cancer, including breast and prostate cancers. The combination of vitamin C and lycopene also helps to prevent the buildup of cholesterol in your bloodstream.
- Beans have a high fiber content that helps to reduce the absorption of both fat and calories from the intestinal tract, not to mention the fact that they help reduce your appetite by filling you up on fewer calories. Beans are also high in potas-

sium and low in sodium, which helps to reduce the risk of high blood pressure and strokes.

• Sweet potatoes are, contrary to popular belief, excellent sources of vitamins and minerals and are considered good carbs. They are a great addition to any weight-loss program because of their high fiber content and their nutritional value. Sweet potatoes are good sources of vitamin C, B-complex vitamins, folic acid, potassium, vitamin A, and beta-carotene. These nutrients, combined with plant sterols found in sweet potatoes, are powerful antioxidants, which can help to lower cholesterol and lower your risk of heart disease. When sweet potatoes are eaten with their skin, they are a good source of both insoluble and soluble fiber.

• Asparagus is an excellent source of potassium, folic acid, beta-carotene, vitamin C, and the antioxidant glutathione, which helps to fight nasty free radicals, which can damage normal cells. Asparagus is a great addition to any diet program, since it is low in calories and high in fiber and nutrients. Steamed asparagus is great eaten alone or in a salad. Leftovers must be refrigerated or frozen quickly, however, to prevent the loss of nutritional value. Asparagus should be lightly steamed or roasted. If boiled too long, most of the nutrients end up in the water.

• Peppers, including red, green, and yellow sweet peppers, are excellent sources of vitamin C, vitamin A, beta-carotene, B-complex vitamins, potassium, and folic acid. They are low in calories and high in fiber, so peppers are excellent foods to add to your weight-loss program. Because they are so flavorful, peppers satisfy your taste buds and help reduce your appetite. Peppers contain antioxidants, which help to prevent blood clots, thereby helping to prevent heart attacks and strokes. Hot peppers have higher quantities of antioxidants than sweet peppers, as well as phytonutrients that assist in preventing certain forms of cancer. Hot peppers contain an ingredient, *capsaicin*, that not only makes them hot and spicy but gives them anti-inflammatory properties that help to relieve the pain of various forms of arthritis and nerve inflammations.

■

PART 3

Shed More Pounds with Protein

Tip 18 Get Lean with Lean Protein

The addition of low-fat protein to your diet short-circuits the appetite control mechanism (appestat) in the brain, making you feel less hungry. Because it takes your body longer to digest protein than it does to digest fat or refined carbohydrates, protein causes a very gradual rise in the blood sugar, which in turn causes a very moderate rise in insulin levels and satisfies your hunger.

Adding healthy protein to your diet is easy. Good sources of healthy, lean protein include:

- Fish, skinless poultry, and very lean meats such as lamb and pork, as opposed to beef, which has an extremely high fat content
- Low-fat dairy products, such as nonfat milk, low-fat or nonfat cheese, and yogurt
- Egg whites
- Vegetable proteins such as nuts, beans, legumes, and tofu

When you are on a low-calorie diet, your body needs more protein for energy production and cell maintenance. Have a small amount of lean protein with each meal to give the body the building blocks it needs for your metabolism. Protein can help to satisfy your hunger significantly longer than high-fat or high refined carbohydrate meals because it takes the body considerably longer to digest and absorb protein than it does for the body to process carbohydrates and fats. Proteins like cheeseburgers, hot dogs, and bacon, however, are unhealthy, high-fat proteins and should be eaten sparingly.

Tip 19 Strike a Healthy Balance

If you combine lean protein with healthy high-fiber complex carbohydrates you will feel satisfied sooner and stay satisfied longer. The more balanced your meal, the less hungry you'll feel after it!

Refined carbohydrates, such as baked goods, white bread, white rice, white potatoes, low-fiber breads and cereals, and sugary desserts are broken down rapidly in the intestinal tract and are just as rapidly absorbed into the bloodstream as glucose. This rapid rise in blood glucose causes a spike in insulin levels and a consequential rapid increase in your hunger.

Protein causes a very gradual rise in the blood sugar, which, in turn, causes a very moderate rise in insulin levels. When you combine high-fiber foods with protein, your body's metabolism processes this fiber-protein combination much more slowly than it would either fiber or protein separately. Your appetite is satisfied more quickly and for a longer period of time, and consequently, you eat fewer calories. The addition of lean protein to your high-fiber snack ensures that you'll be hunger-free until the next meal, without the desire for additional snacking.

In order to balance your meals, stick with complex carbohydrates that are high in fiber and low in sugar. These include fruits, vegetables, whole-grain breads and cereals, whole-grain pastas, nuts, and legumes. Balance these meal plans with small amounts of protein, including lean meats, poultry, fish, egg whites, nuts, beans, tofu, and low-fat dairy products such as milk, cheese, yogurt, cottage cheese, and sour cream.

Tip 20 Boost Energy and Control Hunger with Protein

Protein is found in all of your body's cells. It is the essential nutrient that is responsible for the maintenance and repair of all of your organs, tissues, muscles, brain, and bones. This individual built-in repair kit occurs at the cellular level in our bodies. Protein regulates everything from our blood circulation to our metabolism and our immune system.

All foods are sources of energy; however, protein provides a greater boost in energy levels because it is absorbed slowly and thus produces a constant source of energy. Protein has real energy staying power for your active, healthy lifestyle. Fats and carbohydrates produce quick bursts of energy but do not provide the body with a continuous source of energy, since they are digested and metabolized more quickly than protein. Fats and carbohydrates also tend to be stored as fat in the body for later use.

Individuals who lack sufficient protein in their bodies have weaker immune systems than people who consume adequate protein in their diets. Also, people who are constantly on yo-yo diets where they lose and gain weight back frequently become protein deficient and have weaker immune systems. Researchers have found that yo-yo dieters have about a third fewer killer cells than normal individuals. These so-called killer blood cells are essential for the immune system to function properly.

In order to reap the benefits of protein-rich foods and avoid unnecessary saturated fat, eat lean protein such as lean meats, fish, skinless poultry, seafood, egg whites, low-fat dairy products, legumes, beans, soy foods, and good-fat nuts. Lean proteins are also excellent sources of selenium, which is a mineral that protects the body against dangerous free radicals that can destroy normal cells in the body. These free radicals can damage many different types of cells including connective tissue, which causes joint and muscle inflammation.

High saturated fat protein products like fatty meats, hard cheeses, whole-fat dairy products, whole eggs, mayonnaise, and luncheon and smoked meats including bacon, sausage, and hot dogs are not ideal sources of energy. Even though these products have protein content, this value is offset by their saturated fat content. The saturated fat in these foods does more harm to the body in the form of heart disease, strokes, hypertension, high cholesterol, and some forms of cancer than the protein does good. For this reason, these are called harmful proteins and are not recommended for any healthful weight-loss program.

For appetite control, lean protein tops the charts for staying power. By adding a small portion of lean protein to your meal, you'll control hunger pangs for hours. Lean protein also has the advantage of being lower in calories than many other foods, particularly saturated fat protein products, refined carbohydrates, and other saturated fat foods. Saturated fat protein products defeat the appetite-controlling factor of the protein. The fat content of saturated fat protein foods prevents the brain's appetite control center from shutting down. In other words, soon after you enjoy that cheeseburger, hot dog, or bacon, you'll be hungry again.

How Much Protein Is Enough?

Your body needs between 15 and 30 percent of its total daily calories to come from protein. To determine the number of grams of protein your body needs for a fairly active individual, multiply your body weight in pounds by 0.5. For example, if you weigh 130 pounds, multiply that by 0.5 and you'll find that you need approxi-

mately 65 grams of protein daily for your body to function efficiently. If you're very active, then you multiply your weight in
pounds by 0.7. If you're sedentary, multiply your body weight by
0.4. Eating too much protein, more than 35 percent of your total
daily calories, however, can be dangerous, because it strains the kidneys. This is one of the reasons to steer clear of low-carbohydrate,
high saturated fat protein diets.

Tip 21 Make Smart Protein Choices

With all the diet information out there on what to eat and what not to eat—diets that call for no carbs, diets that call for no fats—it's hard to make heads or tails of what's really good for you. Here are some basic guidelines to help you make good choices that will help you trim down:

Beef

As red meat contains high levels of bad saturated fat, a good rule of thumb is to limit beef intake to no more than once a week.

- When you do eat meat, opt for lean cuts of meat. "Prime grade" meat actually contains the highest amount of saturated fats. "Choice" meat is the next highest in fat content. Choose "Lean" meats or "Select" meats, which have a slightly lower fat content.
- Avoid bacon, sausage, hot dogs, kielbasa, knockwurst, and high-fat lunchmeats, including liverwurst.
- Always trim the fat from meats before cooking.
- Avoid organ meats (brain, liver, kidney, thymus), which are very high in cholesterol and saturated fat.

Poultry

Chicken and turkey are good sources of protein and a low-fat alternative to red meat.

- Always remove the skin before cooking meat, since the fat content of the skin is absorbed during the cooking process.
- Opt for white meat, as it contains less fat than dark meat.
- If possible, choose free-range organic chicken, which does not contain chemicals and hormones and is therefore healthier for you.
- Low-fat turkey breast makes for high-protein, healthy sandwiches or salads.
- Avoid breaded or fried chicken or chicken nuggets, which are particularly high in saturated and trans fat.
- Avoid internal organs, such as liver, which again are very high in cholesterol and saturated fat.

Fish

Fish is an excellent source of protein and contains the added benefit of containing heart-healthy omega-3 fatty acids. Fattier fish like tuna, salmon, sardines, herring, and haddock are particularly high in omega-3 fatty acids. Most fish are low in total saturated fats and cholesterol. Shrimp, lobster, crab, and other shellfish are high in cholesterol; however, shellfish is so low in total fat that its cholesterol content is unlikely to raise your blood cholesterol.

- Always grill, broil, poach, or bake fish without breading. Add spices and lemon to enhance flavor.
- Limit large fish intake, such as shark, swordfish, tuna, and tile fish, since they may be higher in mercury content. This is especially true if you are pregnant or nursing.

Dairy

Dairy products provide your body with two essentials: protein and calcium.

- Drink nonfat or 1 percent milk; 2 percent milk contains almost as much fat as whole milk.
- Choose low-fat cheeses like cottage cheese, goat cheese, skim milk mozzarella, and low-fat Swiss cheeses. Limit your intake of high-fat processed cheeses like American, cheddar, Brie, and Roquefort cheese.
- Butter is very high in saturated fat, and margarine is just as bad for you, since it is high in partially hydrogenated poly-unsaturated fats. There are some newer butter substitutes on the market that are supposed to be heart-friendly. Use them sparingly.
- Yogurt, sour cream, and cream cheese are rich in protein and can be found in low-fat or nonfat varieties. Always add fruit, when possible, to beef up the nutrient content.

Other Protein Sources

Eggs are an excellent source of protein. Egg whites in particular are a great source of protein and don't contain the cholesterol found in egg yolk; however, two to three whole eggs per week are still part of a healthy diet, and the yolk contains many nutrients that are good for you. An egg white or egg substitute omelet is a good alternative to whole eggs. With plenty of fresh veggies, it makes for a health-ful, low-fat, high-protein meal. Be sure to cook it using a sparse amount of olive oil, as opposed to butter or margarine.

Soy milk, tofu, and tempeh all are rich in protein and contain plant nutrients. Many also contain healthy isoflavones, which have estrogen-like qualities and can also have positive effects in meno-pausal symptoms and may help to lower blood fats. The isoflavones in soy help break down fat stored in your body's fat cells and help reduce your risk of heart disease.

Tip 22 Drink Milk for a Double Weight-Loss Benefit

The unique combination of calcium and protein that is present in milk, yogurt, and cheese helps the body to burn fat and store protein. Low-fat dairy products rev up your metabolism, causing your muscles to burn more fat, and block fat storage in your abdomen, thighs, and hips. Taking at least 1,000 milligrams of calcium per day has been shown to reduce the risk of heart attacks and strokes by increasing good (HDL) cholesterol in the bloodstream and decreasing bad (LDL) cholesterol. At the same time, the protein present in milk, yogurt, and cheese replaces the fat stored in cells by providing them with protein, the natural building block to activate all of the body's cells, tissues, and organs' metabolic functions.

Research shows that drinking two glasses of skim milk or eating two cups of yogurt or one serving of low-fat cheese per day may help you lose weight without cutting calories. Several studies have shown that people who regularly drink skim milk and eat yogurt lose an average of a pound and a half per month with no additional change whatsoever in their diets.

Nonfat milk, low-fat cheeses, and nonfat or low-fat yogurt have the same minerals, vitamins, protein, and calcium as whole milk without the added fat content; fat-free milk contains a healthy 220 milligrams of calcium and only 80 calories per glass.

What better snack food could you find than a glass of skim milk that lowers your cholesterol and reduces your waist size at the same time? Or try alternative high-calcium and fat-burning foods such as cheese, tofu, nonfat cottage cheese, spinach, collard greens, and calcium-fortified fruit juices; just be wary of fruit juices with high sugar content.

Tip 23 Beat Nighttime Cravings with Protein

There is a condition called night eating syndrome or NES that is actually a form of an eating disorder. People with NES wake up many times during the night and are unable to fall asleep unless they eat something, usually junk food, that enables them to fall back to sleep. There is another documented night eating disorder that is called sleep-related eating disorder, or SRED. In this condition, people sleepwalk to the kitchen for an eating binge. In both of these conditions, people eat mostly junk food, which can thwart attempts at staying on a balanced nutritious diet. These two types of night eating disorders also undermine good quality sleep. Both of these disorders require treatment by a physician.

These conditions may sound extreme, but there are milder variations of these disorders that can keep many healthy people from continuing on a weight-loss program. People who are under stress may develop some minor form of a night eating disorder that causes them to eat lots of empty calories at bedtime or during the night. Others just develop a habit of night eating that becomes very difficult to break.

Most often these nighttime snacks are junk foods such as cookies, doughnuts, and cakes, which are high in calories, fat, and sugar. This refined carbohydrate fix temporarily raises the blood sugar and causes night eaters to be able to fall asleep. Unfortunately, they are often awakened again by the subsequent drop in blood sugar level that makes them hungry again.

The best remedy for most people who have this milder form of nighttime eating disorder—people who either have difficulty falling asleep or often wake up during the night and can't go back to sleep—is to have a small lean, high-protein snack. For example, a slice of low-fat cheese, handful of nuts, glass of skim or soy milk, a cup of nonfat yogurt, or even a slice of turkey will satisfy that night-time hunger. These lean, high-protein snacks are appetite satisfying, take longer to digest than carbohydrates, and help break the vicious junk-food bingeing cycle of nighttime eating.

As long as you eat a high-protein, low-calorie snack, eating late in the evening will not cause you to gain weight. Calories are calories, no matter when you consume them. Remember, it's the total number of calories consumed in any twenty-four-hour period that counts, not the time that you ate these calories. Nighttime binge eating that involves the consumption of high-calorie, high-fat, high refined sugar snacks, however, will certainly ruin any diet program and may, indeed, cause you to gain weight.

Tip 24 Try These Tasty Protein Snacks

Try these satisfying, high-protein snacks for a healthy way to curb your appetite:

- Smoothie made with 1 cup fat-free milk, ice, and the fruit of your choice: bananas, strawberries, blueberries, and peaches are all great options.
- Whole wheat muffin or scooped-out bagel with one tablespoon low-fat peanut butter, with or without low-sugar jelly or jam.
- One slice whole wheat pizza with light cheese topped with tons of veggies.
- Carrots or celery sticks dipped in salsa or fat-free, low-calorie dressing.
- Two ounces grilled salmon or chicken with mixed greens on the side. Fork-dip your low-calorie dressing of choice as you enjoy this tasty snack.
- Two slices low-fat cheese and tomato melted on a whole wheat muffin or scooped-out bagel.
- One cup low-fat cottage cheese or yogurt with the fruit of your choice.
- Small chicken Caesar salad with Romaine lettuce, low-fat grated Parmesan cheese, one ounce grilled chicken breast, and low-fat Caesar dressing on the side.
- Tuna melt with low-fat cheese on one slice whole wheat bread or half of a whole wheat English muffin with sliced tomato.

- Two slices low-fat turkey breast on one slice whole wheat bread with nonfat or low-fat mayo or mustard and lettuce and tomato.
- One ounce mixed nuts (walnuts, almonds, pecans, peanuts) with one small box raisins.
- Hard-boiled or poached egg on half of a whole wheat English muffin.

PART 4

■

Get the Skinny on Fat

Tip 25 Know the Difference Between Good and Bad Fat

The current guidelines for fat consumption call for no more than 30 percent of your total calories to come from fat. Not only does fat cause people to gain weight, but it also increases the risk for heart disease, stroke, diabetes, and high blood pressure. That's not to say that all fat is bad for you; different foods contain many different types of fats, and some are better for you than others. Here's a general breakdown of the good, not-so-good, bad, and very bad fats.

The Good Fats

Monounsaturated fats are, by far, the best fats. These fats are liquid at room temperature and are found in olive oil, peanut oil, canola oil, most nuts, and avocados. Monounsaturated fats can lower your total blood cholesterol, increase your good HDL cholesterol, and lower your bad LDL cholesterol. To lose weight and stay healthy, you should use them as a substitute for the potentially bad polyunsaturated fats like corn, safflower, sunflower, and cottonseed oils.

The Not-So-Good Fats

Polyunsaturated fats are usually liquid. These fats that are made from vegetables, including sunflower, cottonseed, safflower, and corn oils, are good in small amounts, but turn bad if eaten to excess. In small amounts, polyunsaturated fats help to reduce your cholesterol. However, taken in excess, these polyunsaturated oils can cause an inflammatory reaction in the body's tissues and prevent the immune system from working properly.

The paradoxical good and bad nature of polyunsaturated oils is because they contain omega-6 fatty acids. Omega-6 fatty acids can help to lower blood cholesterol in small amounts; however, when you eat more polyunsaturated fats, you increase the absorption of omega-6 fatty acids in the bloodstream, which causes your cells to absorb more cholesterol and saturated fat. The trick is to eat polyunsaturated fats in moderation.

The Bad Fats

Saturated fats are usually solid and can be considered bad fats as the body uses them to produce LDL cholesterol. LDL cholesterol is what blocks your arteries and causes heart attacks, strokes, and diabetes. Saturated fats come primarily from animal sources that include meats, cheese, butter, milk, and other whole-milk dairy products. Some saturated fats are also found in tropical oils such as coconut, cocoa butter, and palm kernel oils.

Triglycerides are another kind of bad fat. If you eat excess amounts of refined sugar products such as cakes, pies, candy, soda, and baked goods, eat a lot of fattening foods, or drink excessive amounts of alcohol, the liver converts these excess calories into triglycerides. Triglycerides have been implicated in clogging the arteries to the heart and brain.

The Very Bad Fats

Trans fats are very bad fats, probably the worst fats that exist. Trans fats are produced when the polyunsaturated fats in vegetable oils undergo a process called hydrogenation, in which hydrogen atoms are added to the polyunsaturated fat molecules. These very bad trans fats raise your blood levels of bad LDL cholesterol and saturated fat and lower your blood levels of good HDL cholesterol.

Trans fats may also increase the risk of heart attacks, strokes, and diabetes. Several new studies indicate that trans fats can also increase the levels of a cellular component in the body called *tumor necrosis factor*. This cellular component is considered a risk factor for diabetes, insulin resistance, coronary heart disease, heart failure, and certain forms of cancer.

Trans fats are found in foods such as baked goods, cookies, crackers, chips, margarine, and shortening. In order to avoid these really bad fats, avoid all products that say, "hydrogenated" or "partially hydrogenated" on the label. The following is a partial list of foods that contain high levels of trans fats:

Margarine	Crackers, chips, and pretzels
Nondairy creamers	Canned soups and sauces
Packaged cakes and cookies	Fast foods (burgers, fries, and fried foods)
Doughnuts and muffins	Frozen dinners
Cereal and energy bars	Pie, cake, and cookie mixes

Food manufacturers started using hydrogenated fats in place of saturated fats in the mid-1980s, thinking this type of fat would be healthier than saturated fat. Hydrogenated fats were also added to foods to extend the shelf life of certain foods, much like preservatives are added to extend shelf life. It has since been discovered that the trans fats in hydrogenated fats are as bad, if not worse, then saturated fats. For a healthy diet avoid them as much as possible.

Tip 26 Fat Makes You Fat!

While protein and carbohydrates supply your body with 4 calories per gram, one gram of dietary fat supplies your body with 9 calories, making it the most concentrated source of calories. Since fat is a concentrated source of calories, it is the most fattening type of food that we consume.

Weight gain occurs from taking in more calories in the form of dietary fats than are burned off as a fuel for energy. On a low-fat diet, calories are removed from storage in fat cells and added to the fuel mixture of protein and carbohydrate for the production of energy, resulting in steady, permanent weight loss. The equation is simple: less fat taken in results in more stored fat being burned as fuel; more fat taken in results in more fat being stored and less fat being burned, which causes fatty deposits in the abdomen, buttocks, thighs, and hips. In other words, *it's the fat in your diet that makes you fat*!

Since one pound of body fat contains 3,500 calories, it stands to reason that the only way to lose one pound of body weight is to burn 3,500 calories more than you take in. This can only be accomplished by cutting back on the total amount of fat calories in your diet and/or increasing your physical activity. Nothing else works!

Controlling your weight by reducing the amount of saturated fat in your diet has a twofold benefit. First of all, it will help to control and maintain your weight. Second, it will have the beneficial effect of helping to prevent heart attacks and strokes, since these illnesses have been associated with high levels of blood cholesterol, which result from the consumption of saturated fats.

Tip 27 Get the Lowdown on Lipids

The term *lipids* is used to include all fats and fatlike substances that circulate in our bloodstreams. These lipids will not dissolve in water and are therefore called fat-soluble substances. So how do these fats get absorbed into the bloodstream, since the blood is a water-based solution? These lipids have to hook up with certain proteins in our blood so that they can dissolve in water (in this case the blood), and they now become known as lipoproteins, fat and protein combinations. The two main types of lipids in the blood that are combined with proteins are cholesterol and triglycerides. These lipoprotein combinations are classified on the basis of their density in the blood stream.

Cholesterol

Cholesterol is an essential element of all animal cell membranes and forms the structure of the body's hormones and bile acids. However, when cholesterol levels get too high in our bloodstream they can become very dangerous. There are three important types of cholesterol that you have to consider for good health.

- *Total cholesterol* is the total amount of cholesterol circulating in your blood. This is determined by the total amount of cholesterol and fat you eat, combined with the amount of cholesterol manufactured by your liver.
- *LDL cholesterol* (low-density lipoprotein) is referred to as bad cholesterol. This is the type of cholesterol most likely to clog up your arteries and cause heart attacks and strokes. LDL cholesterol comes primarily from eating excess saturated fats and

cholesterol-laden foods. Following a low-fat, high-fiber diet combined with regular exercise can usually lower LDL cholesterol. In many people, however, a high LDL cholesterol level can be genetic and has little or nothing to do with your diet. In these particular cases, someone slipped you a bad cholesterol gene, and oftentimes the LDL can only be lowered by cholesterol-lowering medications prescribed by your physician.

- *HDL cholesterol* (high-density lipoprotein) is called good cholesterol. HDL cholesterol acts opposite to bad cholesterol by helping to prevent the formation of cholesterol deposits in your arteries. It accomplishes this by collecting excess bad cholesterol in the blood before it has a chance to clog up your arteries. It transports this bad cholesterol to the liver, where it is eliminated from the body. Recent medical reports have shown that the HDL cholesterol can actually shovel the bad cholesterol out of the cholesterol deposits (plaques) that have already formed in the arteries. Pretty cool!

Well, how do we get some of this good cholesterol? As always, there's got to be a catch. First and foremost, heredity plays an important role in the body's production of this good cholesterol. Some people have more HDL than others simply because of good genes. Second, cutting saturated fats and cholesterol from our diets has little to do with raising HDL cholesterol. However, adding heart-healthy monounsaturated fats such as olive oil and nuts and the omega-3 fatty acids found in fish such as salmon and tuna has been shown to raise the HDL cholesterol. Regular moderate-intensity exercise, such as walking, can also help to raise the good cholesterol, whereas lack of exercise and smoking will considerably lower the good cholesterol. Individuals who cannot raise their good (HDL) cholesterol and can't lower their bad (LDL) cholesterol by diet and exercise often have to take cholesterol-lowering medications under a doctor's supervision.

Triglycerides

Triglycerides are the major lipids transported in the blood. The triglycerides are the least dense of the fat and protein combinations and are called *very low-density lipoproteins* (VLDL). Triglycerides are important in transferring energy from the food we eat into our bodies' cells, and consequently they help to regulate the cells' metabolism.

Excess amounts of triglycerides in the blood often lead to diabetes, glucose intolerance, obesity, gout, and coronary artery disease. Some cases of high blood triglycerides are genetic, while many others are the result of eating too many refined carbohydrates, sugars, saturated fats, and alcohol. The most important way to control high triglycerides in the blood is to restrict the amount of refined carbohydrates, sugars, and saturated fats you eat and to limit the amount of alcoholic beverages you consume.

A high-fiber diet consisting of whole-grain cereals and breads, beans and other legumes, and fruits and vegetables has been shown to lower high serum triglycerides. A regular aerobic exercise program like walking has also been shown to lower blood triglycerides. However, as with blood cholesterol, there are some cases that cannot be lowered with diet and exercise and have to be treated with medication by a physician.

■ **It's Not Your Willpower, It's Your Triglycerides!**

Several recent studies have shown that it may actually be your triglycerides and not your willpower that are to blame for your desire to overeat. People with high blood triglycerides were shown to have difficulty in curbing their appetites. This appears to be because high blood levels of triglycerides block the formation of an appetite-controlling hormone called *leptin*. This condition sets up a vicious cycle: The more refined sugars and saturated fats you eat, the higher your blood levels of triglycerides become. These high triglycerides shut down the production of the appetite-controlling hormone leptin so you don't feel full when in actuality you are really full. So what do you do next? Eat more refined sugars and saturated fats. The only way to break this overeating cycle is to severely restrict your refined sugars and saturated fats in the first place. Then your triglycerides do not become abnormally elevated and your appetite-controlling hormone leptin is not blocked. Once leptin is released into the blood stream, your appetite will be controlled and you will feel full and stop eating at the appropriate time. Reducing dietary saturated fats helps minimize triglycerides but not as much as reducing your refined sugars and carbs will help with this problem. Cutting down on alcohol and increasing aerobic exercise will also help you reduce your serum triglycerides.

Tip 28 Eat Plenty of Heart-Healthy Omega-3s

The American Institute for Cancer Research has recommended that people eat more foods containing omega-3 fats and fewer food containing omega-6 fats. Omega-3 fats are heart-healthy fats that lower cholesterol and triglyceride levels, prevent blood clots, and help to prevent heart attacks, strokes, and neurological disorders, such as Alzheimer's. Omega-3 fats also have cancer-inhibiting effects against breast and colon cancer. These healthy omega-3 fats are found in fish oils, walnuts, flaxseed, spinach, broccoli, kale, and canola and olive oils.

A Heart-Healthy Catch

Since fish is low in calories and saturated fat, high in protein, and contains the heart-protecting, cancer-fighting benefits of omega-3 fatty acids, it makes for a great diet food.

Even shellfish with its higher content of cholesterol is still an important fat-burning food in your diet program. The low saturated fat content of shellfish offsets the cholesterol that these products contain.

Fish oil has been shown to reduce blood fats and, consequently, slow the formation of deposits of cholesterol in the arteries. In a study at the University of Chicago, monkeys on a diet high in fish oil developed less cholesterol deposits in their arteries than monkeys fed a diet high in saturated fat and coconut oil. The monkeys fed fish oil also had lower total cholesterol and LDL cholesterol levels than the monkeys fed the high saturated fat diet.

Another study conducted at Harvard Medical School appears to indicate that fish oils also have a cancer-inhibiting factor. In a study of rats with breast cancer, fish oils seem to slow the spread of the disease significantly more than diets high in saturated fat or poly-unsaturated fats, and even more than just a low-fat diet. Many recent studies at major universities have also found that the omega-3 oils help to prevent platelet cells in the blood from getting sticky, decreasing the tendency for blood clots to form. Eskimos and the Japanese, who consume lots of fish, don't typically have heart attacks from fat-clogged arteries.

Omega-3 fatty acids found in fish oil also have been found to be essential for brain function. Recent studies have found that a lack of omega-3 fatty acids may be responsible for learning disabilities, memory loss, difficulty concentrating, and certain degenerative dis-eases, including Alzheimer's disease. In a recent study, age-related memory decline was halted or slowed down considerably in women who ate three to four ounces of fish every other day. New evidence has also shown that fish oils may even help in the treatment of major depression and other neurologic and psychiatric disorders.

Eat fish two or three times per week for a healthy heart and a slim body. Salmon, sardines, trout, and herring are particularly high in omega fats. Despite the reports that farmed salmon may contain more chemicals than wild salmon, the American Institute for Can-cer Research says that the benefits of eating fish, whether farmed or wild, outweighs the risks.

Fish and Methyl Mercury

Because some fish are contaminated with high levels of methyl mer-cury, you should get most of your omega-3s by eating a variety of fish known to have low mercury levels. Keep in mind that the health benefits of the nutrients contained in fish will, however, far out-weigh the minimal exposure when consuming fish with low levels of mercury. Also, be particularly careful about taking fish-oil capsules, which may also contain high levels of mercury.

Pile These Fish on Your Plate

According to the FDA, the following fish and shellfish are considered the best fish with the lowest levels of mercury:

1. Cod, catfish, crab, flounder, and sole
2. Grouper, haddock, herring, lobster, and mahi-mahi
3. Ocean perch, oysters, rainbow trout, and salmon
4. Sardines, scallops, tilapia, and farm-raised trout

Eat These Fish Sparingly

The fish that contain the highest levels of mercury are considered the worst fish for human consumption. They are as follows:

1. Mackerel, shark, swordfish, and tile fish
2. Fresh or frozen tuna. Canned tuna, on the other hand, has lower levels of mercury because the tuna used in the canning process are the smaller varieties of fish. Canned tuna labeled "chunk light" tuna has less mercury than "solid albacore" tuna.

Tip 29 Try These Tasty Low-Fat Snacks

There are tons of tasty low-fat snacks out there. Check out these healthy options with their serving sizes.

Grains

When you are in the mood for complex carb, try one of these low-fat options:

- Low-fat, low-sugar cereal bars
- Low-fat whole wheat pretzels (2 small)
- Fat-free baked potato (1 small)
- A handful of corn chips without trans fats
- Rice cakes (2)
- A handful of roasted peanuts in the shell
- Low-fat or fat-free popcorn (1½ cups)
- A handful of sunflower seeds
- 1 small slice of angel food cake
- A few gingersnap cookies
- A handful of high-fiber, low-sugar cereal with or without skim milk
- 1 tablespoon peanut butter on 2 or 3 nonfat crackers

Fruits

Fruits always make for a good high-fiber snack:

- ½ cup raisins, grapes, strawberries, or blueberries
- ½ cup orange, grapefruit, or pineapple wedges

- ⅓ cup dried fruit without added sugar
- 1 sliced banana, pear, or apple
- 3 or 4 pitted prunes

Vegetables

These veggies make for great snacks, alone or dipped in nonfat dip, fat-free dressings, or salsa:

- Celery or carrot sticks (¾ cup)
- Wedge of lettuce, broccoli, or cauliflower (1 cup)
- Sliced cucumbers (½ cup)

Dairy

These dairy options make for a delicious midmorning or midafternoon snack:

- ½ cup nonfat yogurt with or without fruit topping
- 8 ounces skim milk
- ½ cup fat-free cottage cheese or sour cream with or without fruit topping
- ½ cup nonfat, low-sugar ice cream

Sweet Snacks

Let's face it: we all crave something sweet sometimes! Here are some good low-fat snacks to satisfy your sweet tooth:

- 1 low-fat peppermint patty
- ½ cup sherbet, frozen yogurt, or fat-free ice cream
- 1 frozen juice bar
- 6 jelly beans

- 4 sugar-free hard candies (made for diabetics)
- 1 tablespoon fat-free fudge
- Small dollop fat-free whipped cream for fruits

Drinks

These low-fat drinks will quench your thirst without packing on the pounds:

- Decaffeinated diet soda, iced tea, or coffee
- Bottled water
- 8 ounces skim milk
- 8 ounces vegetable juice without added sugar
- 6 ounces nonfat latte or cappuccino with skim milk and no whipped cream. Add small amount of mocha, if desired.
- Protein shake with 1 cup skim milk or yogurt plus fruit of choice, blended with ice and 1 tablespoon wheat germ or whey protein

Tip 30 Know Your High- and Low-Cholesterol Foods

Making heart-healthy choices doesn't have to be complicated. Here are helpful lists of the high-cholesterol foods you should avoid and the low-cholesterol foods to opt for instead:

Avoid these High-Cholesterol Foods

The following foods are high in cholesterol and should be eaten sparingly:

Meat, Fish, and Poultry
- Fatty cuts of beef, pork, ham, veal, and lamb
- Duck
- Goose
- Organ meats (kidney, liver, heart, sweetbread, and brain)
- Luncheon meats and canned meats
- Sausage

Dairy Products
- Whole milk
- Evaporated whole milk
- Cheeses made from whole milk
- Creams (sour, whipped, half-and-half, ice cream, and whole-milk or cream cheeses)
- Egg yolks
- Butter
- Margarine

Bread and Cereal
- Commercial muffins
- Biscuits and butter rolls
- Doughnuts
- Mixes containing whole milk, butter, and eggs
- Corn bread and garlic bread
- Rolls and buns
- Coffee cakes
- Crackers and croissants
- White bread, Italian and French bread
- Granola cereals

Desserts and Snacks
- Commercial pies
- Pastries
- Cookies
- Cake
- Puddings
- Cocoa butter
- Whipped cream
- Ice cream
- Fried foods
- Snack foods
- Coconut
- Potato and corn chips

Opt for These Low-Cholesterol Alternatives

The following foods are low in cholesterol and should be part of your healthy menu.

Meat, Fish, and Poultry
- Chicken and turkey without the skin
- Fresh fish, including flounder, cod, bass, sole, perch, haddock, halibut, salmon, trout, tuna, carp, and pike
- Tuna and salmon packed in water
- Lean ground meat
- Very lean cuts of beef, pork, ham, and veal

Dairy Products
- Nonfat or skim milk
- Low-fat buttermilk
- Evaporated nonfat milk
- Spreads made with plant stanols (Smart Balance or Benecol)
- Egg substitutes
- Low-fat cottage cheese
- Low-fat yogurt
- Cheeses made from skim milk
- Egg whites
- Low-fat cheeses
- Low-fat sour cream

Bread and Cereal
- Whole wheat bread
- Pumpernickel bread
- Rye bread
- Cracked wheat bread
- Bread sticks
- Rice cakes
- Matzo
- Whole-grain and bran hot and cold cereals
- Homemade muffins and biscuits (made with olive or canola oil and egg whites)

- Whole wheat, oat, or bran English muffins
- Nonfat bran muffins
- Whole wheat pita
- Soda crackers

Desserts and Snacks
- Home-baked pastries and pies (made with nonfat milk, liquid olive or canola oil, and egg whites)
- Commercial gelatins
- Cocoa
- Angel food cake
- Sherbet, nonfat ice cream, or frozen yogurt
- Cookies, cakes, and puddings made with monounsaturated oil and nonfat milk
- Honey, marmalade
- Nonfat hard or soft pretzels
- Jelly, jam
- Nuts
- Fruits and vegetables
- Natural peanut butter (made with peanuts only)

Other Low-Cholesterol Foods
- Whole-grain pasta, noodles, and rice
- Vegetables, raw or cooked without sauces, butter, or margarine
- Legumes (chick peas, soybeans, lentils, and baked beans)
- Tea, coffee, and sugar-free carbonated drinks
- Fruits and vegetables

Tip 31 Try These Low-Fat Alternatives for Desserts and Snacks

When you're craving something sweet or a high-fat snack, try these low-fat alternatives:

- Angel food cake with fresh fruit and nonfat whipped cream makes a tasty nonfat dessert. Angel food cake has less than 1.5 grams of fat, as opposed to a slice of cheesecake or chocolate cake that has an exorbitant 14 grams of fat.
- Sherbet, sorbet, frozen fruit bars, and nonfat frozen yogurts are excellent substitutes for your ice cream sweet tooth.
- Salad dressing and mayonnaise are no-no's in a low-fat diet plan. Substitute nonfat dressings or nonfat mayonnaise. Or go without dressing or get the dressing on the side and dip your fork gently into it every two or three bites of salad. That way you'll get the taste without the added fat calories.
- Nonfat popcorn is an excellent low-fat, high-fiber snack. Don't add butter or salt. Use hot-air popper or microwave nonfat varieties.
- Dried or fresh fruits, raisins, peaches, apples, plums, apricots, and bananas all make excellent fat-free snacks.
- Nonfat hard or soft pretzels and rice cakes are excellent low-fat snacks.
- Spread jelly, honey, fruit preserves, and all-fruit jams on your toast instead of margarine or butter.
- Have a baked potato with the skin or nonfat corn chips in place of french fries or potato chips.

Tip 32 Watch Out for Hidden Fats

Fat accounted for approximately 30 percent of Americans' calories in the early 1900s, whereas today more than 40 percent of our calories come from fat. In order to meet the basic nutritional requirements, we need only eat one tablespoon of polyunsaturated oil each day, which supplies the essential fatty acid linoleic acid. This essential fatty acid helps you absorb fat-soluble vitamins. With many eating six to eight times this amount of fat, fat is the primary source of nutritionally empty calories for most people.

Americans have become more conscious of fat consumption in the past ten years; however, only about one-third of the fat we eat is visible fat, such as hard fat on meat, fats and oils used in cooking, and oil-based salad dressings. Most of the fat in our diet, unfortunately, is hidden fat and not as readily noticeable.

Where the Fats Hide

These hidden fats hide in a variety of foods:

- Hard cheeses, cream cheese, deep-fried foods, creamed soups, ice cream, chocolate, nuts, and seeds.
- Processed, prepared foods such as baked goods (pies, cakes, and cookies), processed meats (bologna, hot dogs), snack foods, and instant meals.
- Coffee creamers, whipped toppings
- Spreads and dressings
- Creamed soups or heavy stock soups

Many health food products that are purchased as substitutes for saturated fats themselves have high fat content. Half the calories in nuts and seeds, sesame paste, granola, quiches, and avocados are fat calories. However, nuts and avocados contain the heart-healthy monounsaturated fats.

How to Avoid Hidden Fats

Luckily, these hidden fats aren't too difficult to avoid, just so long as you take these simple steps.

Read Labels Carefully

It's difficult to tell how much fat processed foods contained. At the supermarket, always check the label for the ingredients and remember that the *ingredients are listed in order of their weight.* Therefore, if fat or oil is listed as one of the first two ingredients, then the product is likely to be high in fat, especially if it precedes the flour content; for example, in baked goods. The nutrition facts label will tell you how much total fat and saturated fat is in each serving, and what the serving size is.

Tricky Trans Fats. Trans fat is the worst fat there is. It is produced when unsaturated fat is hydrogenated, turning it into a solid. These worst-for-you trans fats aren't always listed on food labels. To determine whether or not there are trans fats in processed foods, check to see if hydrogenated or partially hydrogenated fats are listed on the ingredients label. In most hydrogenated food products, the trans fat content usually equals one-half the total amount of saturated fat on the label. So, if the label lists 4 grams of saturated fat, you can divide that amount in half, making it 2 grams of trans fat per serving.

Dairy

Low-fat 1 percent milk or skim milk is preferable to any other milk product. Low-fat yogurt, cottage cheese, and ricotta cheese are preferable to other dairy products. Parmesan, feta, and mozzarella cheese made from skim milk have less fat than hard cheeses. Sour cream and sweet cream both are high in fat content and should be avoided.

Use skim milk if you are preparing puddings or custards from a packaged mix. Nonfat ice cream and frozen yogurt have less fat than ice cream and milk shakes. Nonfat and low-fat soft ice creams are available, but watch out for the soft frozen custard, which may contain as much fat as the hard varieties. Buttermilk contains little or no butterfat and can be used in baked goods to add taste and richness.

Alternatives to Fattening Spreads and Dressings

Whipped margarine and butter contain less fat per serving than regular margarine or butter because air or water replaces some of the fat in these products. A tablespoon of mayonnaise or oil may have as many fat calories as a teaspoon of hard fat; however, the softer, more liquid fats are less saturated. It is far better to choose the newer soft spreads that are labeled oil-free, which contain no trans fats.

Salads are fine for a low-fat diet, provided they are made without dressings. Use herbs and spices instead. Occasionally adding lemon juice with the spices will be satisfactory. Monounsaturated olive oil can also be used in limited amounts. If you use a low-calorie salad dressing, make sure that it is also low-fat. The newer nonfat salad dressings are preferable.

Meats

Heavily marbled prime cuts of meats and processed meats are the highest in fat content. Sirloin tip, London broil, and flank steak are leaner than heavily marbled beef. Veal and lamb are leaner than beef. Always buy lean hamburger. Never fry meats; always broil or grill them. Avoid gravies and cream sauces. Instead, make gravy at home after skimming off the fat. Limit your red meat intake to once or twice a week, and always keep portion sizes small.

Fish and Poultry

Tuna and salmon are, surprisingly, among the fattier fishes. However, they contain good-for-you, heart-protective omega-3 fatty acids. Sardines in oil and many forms of smoked fish are also high in fat content. Fresh fish, in particular flounder, cod, halibut, perch, haddock, and sole, have considerably less fat. Tuna packed in water has approximately one-third the fat content of tuna packed in oil. Shellfish are low in saturated fats and will not raise your blood cholesterol when used in moderation.

Poultry should also be broiled or grilled rather than fried. Discard the skin of poultry, preferably before cooking to keep the poultry from absorbing excess saturated fat. Do not use creamed sauces or gravies. Always trim off skin before eating any poultry product.

Baked Goods

Commercially prepared baked goods contain considerable saturated fat. The one exception to this is angel food cake. Fig bars, vanilla wafers, and gingersnaps have less fat than cookies and cakes made with chocolate or cream fillings. Remember to check labels for "partially hydrogenated oils." These contain trans fats, and they can raise your blood cholesterol.

Biscuits, muffins, croissants, and butter rolls are high in fat. English muffins and French or Italian breads are lower in fat content; however, whole wheat, whole-grain breads are best. Bread sticks, matzos, and rice cakes are low-fat substitutes for most potato chips and crackers, which are high in fat content.

Tip 33 Eat Less Fat to Lose More Fat

Next time you reach for the fattening bacon, butter, ice cream, doughnut, cake, or pie, think about this:

Your body metabolizes fats and carbohydrates together in a set ratio governed genetically by your individual body's metabolism. When you restrict the number of fat calories you consume, your body's metabolism automatically controls the amount of refined carbohydrate calories you eat. So, by restricting your fat calories, you crave fewer refined carbohydrates.

The combination of eating less fat and fewer refined carbohydrates makes it next to impossible for you to put on excess weight because you are restricting the total amount of calories that you are eating. So when you eat less fat you're less likely to get fat. Sounds simple? It is!

Tip 34 Tips for Low-Fat Cooking

Even healthy foods can be bad for you if they're not prepared healthfully. In order to make sure that your good intentions become good-for-you meals, follow these simple tips:

- Cook with nonstick pans, as they use less fat than cast iron, copper, or aluminum pans. Opt for nonstick vegetable cooking sprays or use a small amount of olive or canola oil.
- Roast meat, poultry, and fish on a rack so that the fat can drip off during cooking. Baste with defatted broth or vegetable juice to preserve moisture. Never use butter, margarine, shortening, or gravy mixes.
- Trim all visible skin and fat from poultry and meat before cooking.
- Grilled or broiled vegetables, fish, poultry, and lean meats are tasty low-fat dishes. The fat drips away as the foods are cooked.
- Steam vegetables, with or without herbs, in a basket over boiling water. Steaming retains the flavor, color, and nutrients of the vegetables.
- Poaching fish in water at a simmer (just below the boiling point of water) preserves the taste and texture of the fish. Condiments such as garlic or herbs can be added to the liquid to enhance the flavor.
- Stir-frying in a pan or wok is a fast way to cook tasty vegetables, chicken, meats, or fish. Add very small amounts of olive or peanut oil and seasonings, followed by either defatted chicken broth or low-sodium soy sauce.

- For a low-fat sauté, use nonfat vegetable spray or a small amount of wine or defatted broth and mix vegetables and fish, poultry, or meat together in a pan. Add herbs such as thyme, basil, sage, or dill for taste.
- Microwaving food uses the food's own moisture to cook. It's quick and easy, and you don't have to add any fat when microwaving. Almost all foods are microwavable.
- Bake potatoes with the skin for a high-fiber, low-fat, and filling food. Peeling a potato before cooking it removes more than 25 percent of its nutrients and 35 to 40 percent of its fiber. If you have a craving for french fries, you can prepare a low-fat version by slicing potatoes, spraying with nonfat vegetable spray, and baking for 20 to 30 minutes at approximately 350°, or microwaving for 3 to 5 minutes. Remember to keep your portion size small.
- Don't salt poultry, fish, or meat before cooking, as it causes the food to lose a good portion of its vitamin and mineral content during the cooking process.
- On pasta nights, opt for thin pastas such as spaghetti (angel hair/cappellini). Wider pastas are often higher in fat because they are made with eggs. Buy whole-grain pasta or spinach noodles for their high fiber content. Stick to tomato and marinara sauces, or seafood-based sauces without cream.
- Soups and stews can be loaded with hidden fats. Refrigerate them overnight after preparing and skim off the layer of fat that rises to the surface. You'll be removing more than three-quarters of the fat contained in these products. Choose soups loaded with vegetables and beans, and avoid any soups that are cream-based.

PART 5

Power Foods to Put on Your Plate

Tip 35 Eat Five Fruits and Vegetables a Day

We've all heard that an apple a day keeps the doctor away, but the nutritional value and high fiber content in fruits and vegetables are better for you than you might think. Fruits and vegetables are low in fat, and they add flavor and variety to your diet. They contain fiber, vitamins, minerals, phytonutrients, and many beneficial compounds that prevent cardiovascular disease, stroke, cancer, diabetes, or high cholesterol. The nutrients in fruits and vegetables have been associated with a lower risk of heart disease and a lower risk of stroke.

Fruits are high in fiber and low in calories. They satisfy your hunger by taking longer to consume, and they promote good bowel health by providing adequate fiber, which in turn reduces your appetite. Fruits are not only low-fat, low-calorie foods, but they are especially rich in potassium, an essential element, which appears to have blood pressure lowering properties.

Fruits are also good sources of pectin, a soluble fiber found in many fruits and vegetables. This particular type of fiber helps to lower blood cholesterol. Many fruits also contain vitamin C, which helps the pectin lower cholesterol even more than pectin alone. Vitamin C also is important in boosting our immune system and has cancer-inhibiting factors built into its structure.

Vegetables are low in calories, high in fiber, contain no fat, and are great foods for weight loss and weight maintenance. Vegetables of the cabbage family such as broccoli, cauliflower, spinach, brussels sprouts, and squash are also high in both vitamin A and C and rich in cancer-fighting phytonutrients. Many vegetables are good sources of potassium, including sweet potatoes, squash, spinach, beets, tomatoes, and green peppers. Boiling destroys 35 to 40 percent or more of the potassium in vegetables, however, so remember to eat more raw vegetables and steam or microwave vegetables rather than boil them in order to reduce potassium loss.

Carrots and dark green leafy vegetables contain beta-carotene and other carotenes, which are chemical precursors to vitamin A. Vitamin A inhibits compounds in the body called free radicals, which may cause normal cells to turn cancerous. Vitamin A also maintains the integrity of the lungs and the intestinal tract.

■ Beta-Carotene's Cancer-Protective Effect

Beta-carotene appears to have a protective effect against both lung and colon cancer. A recent study conducted at the New York State University in Buffalo found that people with lung cancer had significantly lower blood levels of beta-carotene than did people who were free of the disease. Similar studies have shown that patients with colon cancer also have lower levels of beta-carotene than do healthy individuals.

Five a Day Help Reduce Your Risk of Stroke

The nutrients in fruits and vegetables, such as dietary fiber and antioxidants, are associated with a lower risk of heart disease; a recent study has shown that eating five servings of fruits and vegetables a day translates into a 35 percent reduction in stroke risk. This study, reported in the *Journal of the American Medical Association*, also indicates that each increment of one serving of fruit or vegetables per day was associated with a 7 percent reduction for risk of ischemic stroke in women and men.

The consumption of a variety of vegetables and fruits, such as cruciferous vegetables like broccoli and cabbage, green leafy vegetables, citrus fruits, or vitamin C rich fruits and vegetables resulted in the largest decrease in risk (*JAMA* 282, no. 13; October 6, 1999). All the more reason to eat five fruits and vegetables a day!

Tip 36 Add Some Color to Your Diet!

In addition to being naturally low in calories and high in fiber, colorful fruits and vegetables contain cancer-fighting substances and provide your body with nutritious, disease-preventing vitamins and minerals. Each colored fruit or vegetable contains a different phytochemical, or plant-based chemical, that can decrease the risk of certain types of cancer. For maximum health benefits, you should eat a variety of vegetables and fruits of different colors. Your goal should be to eat at least four or five servings of variously colored fruits or vegetables per day.

A Full Spectrum of Health Benefits

The following is a list of some of the phytochemicals present in fruits and vegetables that can reduce your risks of cancer and heart disease:

Lycopene

A carotenoid, or plant pigment, in the same family as beta-carotene, lycopene gives many fruits and vegetables, including tomatoes, their deep red color. Lycopene has powerful antioxidant properties that have been shown to fight different forms of cancer. According to the American Institute for Cancer Research, fruits and vegetables that contain lycopene, particularly tomatoes, may help to prevent prostate cancer, as well as colon, stomach, lung, esophageal, and pancreatic cancers. Lycopene has also been linked with a lower risk of heart attacks secondary to coronary artery disease.

Beta-carotene

This powerful antioxidant with cancer-fighting properties is found in sweet potatoes, which are also high in dietary fiber, as well as vitamins C and E. Dark green leafy vegetables such as spinach, kale, bok choy, and other greens are great sources of beta-carotene. Orange and deep yellow fruits and vegetables such as pumpkins, papaya, apricots, cantaloupe, mango, winter squash, and carrots also have considerable amounts of beta-carotene.

Flavonoids

This group of phytochemicals is found in a variety of fruits, vegetables, and grains. For instance, grapes contain a substance called transresveratrol, which is found primarily in the grape's skin. Resveratrol, which is also present in grape juice and red wine, has been shown to be instrumental in fighting cancer of the colon, liver, and breast. Resveratrol inhibits the growth of cancer by preventing the start of DNA damage in a cell and the transformation of a normal cell into a cancerous cell. It also helps to inhibit the growth and spread of tumor cells. Recent medical research indicates that resveratrol has cardioprotective properties as well.

Ellagic Acid

This acid, present in many types of fruits, vegetables, and grains, appears to reduce the DNA damage caused by carcinogens such as tobacco smoke and air pollution. Berries contain high amounts of ellagic acid, and as little as one cup of raspberries or blueberries slowed the growth of abnormal colon cells in humans and, in some cases, prevented or destroyed the development of cells that were infected with the human papillomavirus (HPV), which can cause cervical cancer. This particular cancer-fighting agent has also been demonstrated to have similar effects on the cancer cells of the breast and pancreas in animal testing.

Allyl Sulfides

Members of the allium family of plants contain compounds known as allyl sulfides that are instrumental in activating enzymes in the body that break down certain cancer-causing substances and increase the body's ability to excrete them. Examples of the allium family include garlic, onions, shallots, and leeks. Many studies have shown that people who eat lots of garlic have less cancer of the stomach and colon and that garlic inhibits the growth of new cancer cells.

Indoles

Cruciferous vegetables get their name from their four-petaled flowers, which resemble crosses, and include broccoli, cabbage, cauliflower, and brussels sprouts. Vegetables in this family contain indoles, phytonutrients that help to fight cancer. Studies have shown that people who eat an abundance of cruciferous vegetables, particularly broccoli, have a reduced incidence of many types of cancer, including cancer of the colon, bladder, prostate, esophagus, lung, breast, cervix, and larynx.

Anthocyanins

These are plant pigments present in cherries, purple grapes and purple grape juice, raspberries, and strawberries that help to protect against heart disease.

Carotenoids

These are antioxidant plant pigments that are converted to vitamin A by the body and include beta-carotene, lutein, and zeaxanthin. Carotenoids reduce the risk of age-related macular degeneration that leads to blindness. Green beans, collard, kale, mustard, turnip, Romaine and other dark lettuces, seaweed, spinach, and winter squash are important sources of lutein and zeaxanthin.

Isoflavones

The plant chemicals known as isoflavones act as weak estrogens (phytoestrogens). Eating approximately 100 milligrams of iso-flavones daily can improve bone density. Good sources of isoflavones are soy milk, soy protein, tofu, and textured vegetable proteins.

Folic Acid

One of the B vitamins, folic acid helps prevent birth defects and lowers levels of homocysteine, which is an amino acid related to folic acid that has been linked to heart disease. Excellent sources of folic acid include oranges, broccoli, Romaine and other dark lettuces, and spinach.

As you can see, phytochemicals are a rainbow of multiple colors, and each of these colorful fruits and vegetables offers a full spectrum of disease prevention.

Tip 37 Eat These Top Twenty Antioxidant Foods

Antioxidants are wonderful chemicals that help neutralize the free radicals that result when your body converts oxygen into energy. If free radicals aren't neutralized, they have the potential to cause a condition called *oxidative stress*, or an imbalance between the factors that cause oxidation and the factors that inhibit oxidation. Free radicals can also cause cell damage that makes the body's metabolic system and the organs' systems break down.

For a tasty fix of healthy antioxidants, try these top twenty antioxidant-containing foods:

Fruits	Veggies
Apples	Broccoli
Blueberries	Bok choy
Blackberries	Cabbage
Cherries	Carrots
Cranberries	Garlic
Prunes	Kale
Purple grapes	Spinach
Raisins	Squash
Raspberries	Sweet potatoes
Strawberries	
Tomatoes	

Blueberries May Reverse the Aging Process

Blueberries are chock-full of antioxidants and fiber. They are also low in sugar and calories. Many studies have shown that among all the fruits and vegetables, the antioxidant benefits of blueberries are the greatest. New research has indicated that women on antioxidant-rich diets showed fewer age-related disorders than those on a standard diet. The studies showed that among all the fruits and vegetables, the benefits were greatest with blueberries, which reversed age-related effects, for example, loss of balance and lack of coordination. They also discovered that blueberry extract had the greatest effect in reversing aging decline.

Previous studies have shown that both strawberries and spinach extract can also help to prevent the onset of age-related defects. However, the greatest effect was shown in patients who ate blueberries. Phytonutrients in blueberries, particularly flavonoids and beta-carotene, seem to have an anti-inflammatory effect, which may even help in the prevention of Alzheimer's disease (*The Journal of Neuroscience* 19: 8114–8121; September 15, 1999).

Protect Your Eyesight with Kale and Spinach

Kale and spinach are two vegetables rich in antioxidants lutein and zeaxanthin that help protect against age-related cataracts and macular degeneration, one of the leading causes of blindness. Romaine lettuce, broccoli, collards, turnip greens, and corn are also high in these vision-protecting antioxidants.

Broccoli: Beats the Big Three

Scientists have known for years that eating dark green leafy vegetables can cut your risk of developing certain forms of cancer. A new medical study, however, has shown that eating broccoli and broccoli sprouts may also reduce your risk of heart disease, high blood pressure, and stroke as well. Broccoli and broccoli sprouts have high concentrations of the antioxidant *glucoraphanin*, which has been shown to boost the body's defense mechanism against cancer-forming free radicals.

A recent study by the University of Saskatchewan reported that laboratory animals prone to high blood pressure that were fed broccoli sprouts with high levels of glucoraphanin had lower blood pressure, less inflammation, a stronger immune system, and less incidence of heart disease and strokes. Newer studies have reported similar findings in humans who consumed abundant amounts of these leafy, bushy, dark green vegetables.

■ More Antioxidant-Rich Cancer Fighters

For other antioxidant-rich foods that may help decrease the likelihood of developing cancer, try soybeans, ginger, licorice, celery, cilantro, parsley, parsnips, onions, brussels sprouts, and mushrooms.

Tip 38 Drink the Ultimate Diet Food

Two-thirds of our body is made up of water. Water is essential for our very existence because it transports nutrients and oxygen though the bloodstream to all of our body's cells and removes toxins and waste products from our body's tissues. Water regulates our body's temperature and metabolism and aids in the digestion of all of the food we ingest. Water also provides the lubrication that makes our muscles and joints move efficiently and effortlessly.

Drinking water fuels the body's energy level because the body's metabolic process requires a constant supply of water to function properly and efficiently. Your body actually loses water all of the time just by the daily activity of living, whether you're active or sedentary. So you need to replenish your body with water constantly in order to replenish those losses.

Water is also the ultimate diet food because it contains no calories and satisfies your hunger quickly. Many people who think they're hungry are in fact actually dehydrated. When your stomach is empty it is often the result of a lack of both food and water. Starting every meal with a glass of water is the best way to satisfy your appetite before you eat, and it will keep you from eating excess calories at each meal. Water is also the best way to keep your appetite in check between meals.

Most studies show that for good health you should drink between eight to ten cups of water daily. A good rule of thumb is to drink half your weight in ounces daily. For example, if you weigh 140 pounds, you should drink seventy ounces or approximately nine cups of water daily. This daily amount of water is the amount that is needed just for normal daily hydration. For exercise, the amount of additional water needed for proper hydration increases with the level of intensity of the activity. To prevent dehydration, you should drink one and a half cups of water thirty minutes before you exercise. Drink an additional cup of water for each fifteen minutes that you exercise moderately and two cups of water for each fifteen minutes of severe exercise where you perspire freely.

The best sources of water are portable bottled water or tap water. Stay away from caffeine whenever possible because it can speed up your metabolism and dehydrate you. Alcohol dehydrates you as well. Fruits, vegetables, soups, Jell-O, yogurt, and other liquid foods all count toward your daily water requirements. Several servings of fruits and vegetables can provide as much as two to three cups of water daily.

Tip 39 Take These High-Energy Foods for a Spin

Here are some great go-to foods for a nutritious burst of energy:

Oatmeal

Oatmeal is high in fiber, low in fat, and low in calories. Oatmeal helps to prevent heart disease by lowering your bad cholesterol (LDL) and increasing your good cholesterol (HDL). Many studies have confirmed these findings, and oatmeal is an essential heart-protecting good food. Top your oatmeal off with bananas or berries to increase the flavor and to add extra nutrients and antioxidants to a delicious breakfast snack. Add nonfat milk to your oatmeal for the calcium that your body needs without the added fat present in whole or low-fat milk.

Yogurt

Calcium-rich yogurt keeps your bones strong and helps to fight off infection by boosting your immune system. The live bacilli in yogurt help to keep your intestinal tract in tip-top shape. All of these benefits are afforded you with either nonfat or low-fat yogurt. You don't need the extra fat content of whole-milk yogurt for it to do its magic. Add fruit to beef up the flavor, nutrition, and antioxidant value.

Spinach: The Health Powerhouse

If you're looking for a vegetable with super healing powers, try spinach. It's packed with vitamins, minerals, and antioxidants including beta- and alpha-carotenes, lutein, zeaxanthin, potassium, magnesium, vitamin K, and folic acid that will protect you from many diseases. Spinach is also a great way to increase your fiber and vitamin C intake. Recent studies have found that eating spinach may lower your risk of strokes, colon cancer, cataracts, heart disease, osteoporosis, hip fractures, memory loss, Alzheimer's disease, depression, and even birth defects.

The disease-fighting properties in spinach are better absorbed when spinach is cooked with a little olive oil. Sautéed with olive oil and a touch of garlic, spinach makes a great side dish. Fresh spinach can be used in salads or sandwiches instead of boring lettuce.

Canned Salmon, Tuna, or Sardines

These three fishes are a great way to increase your essential, heart-healing, inflammation-fighting omega-3 fatty acids. They also provide extra calcium and protein. Add any one to a whole wheat sandwich with onions, lettuce, tomato, and Dijon mustard, and you have a very tasty lunch. Or just add them to a big tossed salad. The ones packed in water are significantly lower in fat; however, if you like the taste of the oil, make sure you drain the can completely of oil and dry the fish off on a paper towel. You will still be getting the yummy taste of the oil and all of the wonderful benefits of the omega-3 fatty acids.

Tip 40 Eat Foods with Incredible Crunch

Foods that require a good bit of chewing are excellent diet foods, since they take time to chew, and consequently the brain's appestat, or appetite regulating mechanism, is satisfied long before you've had a chance to consume too many calories. Many crunchable foods are high in fiber, so in addition to taking a longer time to eat than comparably sized low-fiber foods they have a ton of nutritional advantages as well. And the high fiber content of crunchy fruits and vegetables produces bulk in the stomach, making you feel fuller faster and stay satisfied longer.

An Apple a Day

There are tons of great options out there for low-calorie, high-fiber snacks with a waist-friendly crunch. Here are some favorites for you to try:

- An apple a day not only keeps the doctor away, but it also keeps the fat away from your body. Apples are high in fiber and are one of the best diet foods.
- Corn is a tasty vegetable that packs a powerful crunch. Try it on the cob, or sprinkle the kernels in a salad for color and flavor.
- The crunch of celery makes for a great midday snack. For a protein treat, spread some low-fat peanut butter on a stalk and crunch away.
- In addition to being a crunchy, high-fiber food, carrots provide your body with cancer-fighting antioxidant beta-carotene and essential vitamins C and E. Add them to your

salad or try dipping them in low-fat dressing or fat-free salsa for a snack.

- Cucumbers are a refreshing and crunchy vegetable that is great alone or on a salad. Next time you feel like snacking, do yourself a favor by spearing a cucumber and dipping it in low-fat salad dressing for a healthy treat.
- Cauliflower, broccoli, string beans, or radishes make for fabulously crunchy additions to your salad, or a great midday snack. They'll satisfy your mouth while satisfying your hunger.

Tip 41 Eat These Power Fruits, Veggies, and Nutrients

There is a group of foods that deliver more nutrition per calorie than others that I like to call Power Foods. These foods are not only packed with vitamins but contain many different types of unique nutrients such as phytonutrients, flavonoids, monounsaturated fats, omega-3 fatty acids, complex carbohydrates, proteins, minerals, fiber, and a whole host of nutrition-boosting compounds. Try adding these healthy, energy-boosting foods to your diet:

Whole Grains

Whole-grain breads and cereals, especially those that contain bran, are excellent sources of fiber, B vitamins, and minerals including zinc, iron, and magnesium. All whole-grain foods help to reduce your appetite because of their high insoluble fiber content. Oats are particularly high in soluble fiber, which helps to clean out the fat in your blood vessels by increasing the good HDL cholesterol and sweeping the bad LDL cholesterol out of the bloodstream.

Vegetables

Vegetables are a great source of a variety of essential vitamins and nutrients. Go for these green leafy, cruciferous, or orange veggies:

Green Leafy Vegetables
Green leafy vegetables include spinach, Romaine and other dark lettuces, kale, bok choy, chard, collard greens, and seaweed. These foods are excellent sources of beta-carotene, B-complex vitamins, folic acid, and antioxidants known as carotenoids. These nutrients

and antioxidants help to reduce the risk of certain eye and neurological disorders and also help to prevent heart disease and certain forms of cancer.

Cruciferous Vegetables

Cruciferous vegetables include broccoli, cabbage, and cauliflower. They are an excellent source of complex carbohydrates and dietary fiber. Several studies have shown that people who eat an abundance of cruciferous vegetables have a reduced incidence of several types of cancer. These vegetables are good sources of beta-carotene and B-complex vitamins.

Orange Vegetables

Orange vegetables, including carrots, sweet potatoes, pumpkins, butternut squash, winter squash, and cantaloupe, are loaded with cancer-fighting antioxidants beta-carotene and vitamins C and E.

Fruits

In addition to tasting great and adding color to your diet, these fruits are chock-full of essential vitamins and nutrients:

Tomatoes

Tomatoes are unique in their ability to produce an amino acid called carnitine, which increases the body's basal metabolic rate to help the body burn fat at a faster rate. Tomatoes also contain abundant amounts of vitamin C and an important antioxidant called lycopene, which helps to reduce the risk of several types of cancer. Lycopene is released in higher amounts when tomatoes are cooked.

Berries

Berries are great eaten alone, sprinkled on your morning cereal, or as a tasty smoothie ingredient. Carotenoids, other antioxidants, and vitamin C, which help counteract many chemical processes that contribute to the formation of cancer, are all found in various berries. Cranberries are low in calories and contain vitamin C and antioxidants called procyanidins that keep the urinary tract healthy. Strawberries and raspberries are packed with antioxidants, carotenoids, and vitamin C. Purple grapes contain vitamin C, potassium, and a flavonoid called transresveratrol, which helps to reduce the risk of heart disease. Blueberries are packed with antioxidants and fiber and are low in sugar and calories. The antioxidants in blueberries help neutralize dangerous free radicals and have a significant effect on reversing age-related disorders. (See Tip 37.)

Citrus Fruits

Citrus fruits such as oranges, lemons, and tangerines contain antioxidants and are high in vitamin C, potassium, and folic acid. They provide the body with essential nutrients.

Grapefruit. Grapefruit in particular contains high levels of potassium, vitamin C, beta-carotene, and the antioxidant lycopene, which has been shown to reduce the risk of both breast and prostate cancers. Grapefruits also contain bioflavonoids, which appear to protect against heart disease. They also contain phenolic acid, which can block nitrosamines, which are cancer-causing chemicals found in many smoked foods.

Grapefruits are a great addition to any weight-reduction program, since they are low in calories and high in fiber. The only precaution is that people who are on cholesterol-lowering drugs called statins should be careful about drinking grapefruit juice with these medications. Grapefruit juice appears to slow the natural breakdown of these drugs in the bloodstream, causing higher than expected levels of these medications to stay active in the blood for longer periods of time. It is important for anyone who is taking statin medication to check with his or her doctor before combining grapefruit with these cholesterol-lowering drugs.

Oranges. Oranges protect your heart and fight cancer. In a recent study, it was shown that oranges boost the good HDL cholesterol, in addition to providing vitamin C, folic acid, and numerous flavonoids. These compounds are thought to prevent cholesterol oxidation, which has been linked to a reduced risk of coronary events.

An orange or two a day will keep atherosclerosis away. Researchers have found that citrus fruits, in particular oranges, help decrease the likelihood of developing cancer. These researchers found that animals that ate oranges for several months were 25 percent less likely to develop early colon cancer than animals given only water. Compounds such as liminoids in oranges seem to alter the characteristics of the colon lining, discouraging cancer growth. These researchers speculate that oranges may also help to suppress breast cancer, prostate, and lung cancer.

Legumes

Legumes such as beans and lentils are high in fiber and are excellent sources of protein, without the fat found in meats and dairy products. The high fiber content of beans and lentils helps to reduce the absorption of saturated fat, cholesterol, and calories from the intestinal tract, reduces your appetite, and may reduce the risk of heart disease. These foods are also rich in potassium, iron, zinc, B_6, and folic acid.

Nuts and Seeds

Nuts, particularly walnuts and almonds, are rich in heart-healthy monounsaturated fats and are excellent sources of fiber and protein. Nuts are also a great source of folic acid, vitamin D, copper, and magnesium. Seeds like flaxseed, sunflower seeds, and pumpkin seeds contain phytoestrogens called *lignans*, which have a balancing effect on the body's hormones as well as antioxidant properties. Seeds are also abundant sources of protein, iron, vitamin E, and phosphorus.

Omega-3 Fatty Acids

Seafood, in particular salmon, trout, and tuna, are good sources of protein, nutrients, and omega-3 fatty acids. Omega-3 fatty acids may help to reduce the risk of heart disease and prevent the development of certain forms of cancer. Flaxseed oil is another excellent source of omega-3 fatty acids.

Monounsaturated Fats

Olive oil, olives, canola oil, and peanut oil, as well as nuts and avocados, contain heart-healthy monounsaturated fats. These fats help to reduce the bad LDL cholesterol and raise the good HDL cholesterol and can help to offset the bad effects of eating too many omega-6 fatty acids that are present in processed foods.

Tip 42 Pile on the Soy!

Soybeans help you lose weight and reduce the risk of cardiovascular disease, in addition to other health benefits. Soy contains natural phytonutrients called *isoflavones* that break down the fat stored in your body's fat cells. Several studies have confirmed that the consumption of soy products on a regular basis helps dieters burn fat and lose weight without any other alteration in their diets. These isoflavones have also been shown to reduce the incidence of heart disease by breaking down saturated fat in your blood, and thus lowering the bad LDL cholesterol. Clinical trials showed a significantly lower incidence of coronary heart disease in patients with a high soy intake.

In a related study, soy supplements were shown to cut the risk of developing colon cancer in half. Soy supplements also decreased the relative risk of having a recurrence of colon cancer in high-risk subjects. This study was reported at the annual conference of the American Institute for Cancer Research. High soy intake may be able to delay the onset of colon cancer in those at risk, or may lead to more cancer-free years in those whose initial cancer was surgically removed. The isoflavones in soy can offset some of the adverse effects of estrogen on the body. By decreasing meat, increasing soy intake, and increasing fiber, the body is less likely to develop estrogen-related uterine and breast tumors.

Soybeans can be found in many different foods, including soy beverages, tofu, tempeh, soy-based meat substitutes, soy yogurt, and some baked goods. However, such soy-rich foods should contain at least 6.5 grams of soy protein and less than 3 grams of total fat per serving, with less than 1 gram of saturated fat per serving, to qualify as a heart-healthy food. One-half cup of edamame (cooked soybeans) contains 4 grams of fiber. Soy products are good for the heart and great for your figure!

Tip 43 Pop a Healthy, Low-Calorie Snack

Without the added salt, oil, and butter, popcorn is probably one of the best diet snacks available because it is low in calories and cholesterol and high in fiber. It consequently fills you up without adding extra calories and provides 2 grams of fiber per cup with only 25 calories.

The electric hot-air popper is by far the most efficient way to prepare popcorn because it uses no oil, there are no added fats, and no cleanup is necessary. Hot-air poppers can produce great quantities of popcorn in a relatively short time. This electric appliance is a must for your low-cholesterol, high-fiber, low-calorie diet. Most microwavable popcorns contain considerable fat; however, several newer products are available in low-fat varieties. Always check the label.

Here are some combinations that can be used with popcorn to add flavor and variety to this low-calorie snack:

- **Popcorn croutons.** Popcorn can be used in salads and soups in place of croutons.
- **Popcorn and peanuts.** Popcorn and peanuts (unsalted, dry-roasted peanuts) can be an excellent evening snack with a glass of diet soda. For a sweet and healthy kick, toss some raisins into the mix.
- **Apple and popcorn.** Slices of apple mixed with popcorn make an ideal snack.

Be creative with popcorn. Apple popcorn crisp, parmesan popcorn, cheddar cheese popcorn, garlic popcorn, peanut butter popcorn balls, raisin or cinnamon popcorn, and fruit popcorn balls are some examples. Mix the ingredients in after making the popcorn, and only add small amounts of sugar and fats to your snack.

Tip 44   Go Nuts for Nuts

Recent studies have shown both the health benefits and the weight-reduction properties of nuts. Nuts are chock-full of nutrition. They contain folic acid, vitamin D, copper, magnesium, fiber, and healthy monounsaturated fats. Nuts are also packed with protein, which is good for you and acts as a natural appetite suppressant because it is digested slowly and is subsequently slowly absorbed into the bloodstream. Almost all of the energy contained in the protein you eat is burned as fuel for your body's metabolic functions; hardly any of the calories contained in dietary protein are converted into fat storage. Therefore, nuts are not only good for you, but they don't put on extra weight, providing you limit the amount you consume.

Consuming four to five servings of nuts per week has been shown to reduce the risk of coronary heart disease by as much as 50 percent. Nuts have also been shown to decrease total cholesterol by 5 to 10 percent and LDL cholesterol by 15 to 20 percent. This is all thanks to the monounsaturated fats that nuts contain that have heart-protective properties and help to suppress your appetite so that you eat less. The monounsaturated fats block the production and absorption of bad LDL cholesterol; less bad cholesterol in the bloodstream equals less heart disease. These monounsaturated fats can also help to reduce blood pressure by retaining your blood vessels' natural elasticity, which keeps the arteries open.

Nuts, particularly walnuts and almonds, cause the brain to release a hormone called *cholecystokinin*, which actually shuts down the appetite control mechanism in the brain and prevents hunger. Two ounces of almonds will release this appetite-suppressing hormone. And what's more, nuts taste good. Just remember to limit portion size to a handful.

The Best Nuts

The following are the best nuts, with serving sizes and nutrition information.

- Almonds: ½ ounce, or 12 nuts (80 calories, 7 grams of fat, and high in protein, magnesium, calcium, and vitamin E)
- Walnuts: ½ ounce, or 7 nuts (90 calories, 9 grams of fat, and high in omega-3 fatty acids and alpha-linoleic acid)
- Cashews: ½ ounce, or 10 nuts (80 calories, 6 grams of fat, and high in copper, magnesium, and iron)
- Hazelnuts: ½ ounce, or 10 nuts (85 calories, 8 grams of fat, and high in vitamin E, fiber, and iron)

Walnuts

The beneficial components of walnuts include L-arginine, which dilates the arteries and may therefore have cardioprotective benefits. Walnuts also contain fiber, folic acid, gamma-tocopherol, and other antioxidants that also help to prevent hardening of the arteries.

A study published in the March 2002 issue of *Journal of Nutrition* indicated that of all edible plants, walnuts have one of the highest concentrations of antioxidants. In a study reported in the April 6, 2004, issue of *Circulation*, Dr. Emilio Ros from the Hospital Clinic of Barcelona, Spain, said, "This is the first time a whole food, not its isolated components, has shown this beneficial effect on vascular health." He further stated that "Walnuts differ from all other nuts because of their high content of alpha-linolenic acid (ALA), a plant-based omega-3 fatty acid, which may provide additional heart-protective properties."

The Good Nuts

Other nuts are also good for you, though not as beneficial as the "best" nuts. The "good" nuts, with serving sizes and nutrition information, are as follows:

- Peanuts: ½ ounce, or 20 nuts (80 calories, 7 grams of fat, and high in protein, iron, and folate)
- Pecans: ½ ounce, or 10 nuts (93 calories, 10.2 grams of fat, and high in fiber, copper, and zinc)
- Pistachios: ½ ounce, or 23 nuts (78 calories, 6.3 grams of fat, and high in potassium, fiber, and protein)

The Not-So-Good Nuts

The nuts in the following list should be eaten sparingly:

- Macadamias: ½ ounce, or 5 nuts (102 calories, 10.5 grams of fat; much too high in total fat and calories)
- Chestnuts: ½ ounce, or 2 nuts (55 calories, 0.5 gram of fat, and some folate; even though they are low in calories and fat, chestnuts have no heart health nutritious benefits)
- Brazil nuts: ½ ounce, or 4 nuts (90 calories, 9.5 grams of fat, and moderate levels of selenium and magnesium; there have been cases of Brazil nuts causing sickness due to contaminants, and these nuts are not recommended healthy nuts)

Tip 45 Drink Green Tea

Recent studies point to green tea as a natural way to help you lose weight and help lower your blood pressure. A study from London found that drinking green tea on a daily basis was helpful in weight reduction by a process known as thermogenesis. Thermogenesis is controlled by the sympathetic nervous system and increases the basal metabolic energy rate, thus causing fat oxidation. In other words, it causes the burning of fat in the body. Plant compounds in tea, particularly caffeine and catechins, work together to increase thermogenesis. A similar study reported in the *American Journal of Clinical Nutrition* showed that the daily consumption of two cups of green tea increased the basal metabolic rate 4 percent over a twenty-four-hour period. Unlike drugs such as ephedrine, green tea extracts do not increase the heart rate and are not associated with harmful cardiovascular effects.

Recent studies also indicate that the chemical compounds in green tea can also help lower your cholesterol. In a study published in the September 2004 issue of the *Archives of Internal Medicine*, it was reported that people who regularly drank green tea had a significant reduction in blood pressure. The study showed that individuals who consumed one or two cups of green tea or oolong tea daily for at least one year reduced their risk of hypertension by at least 65 percent. Several previous studies reported by Taiwan's National Science Council reported these same blood pressure lowering effects of drinking green tea.

It is important to note that most of these studies are preliminary and that many people have sensitivities to caffeine and other plant compounds present in tea, particularly green tea. If you are already a tea drinker and have previously suffered no ill effects, then one to two cups of green tea a day may help with your weight-loss program. Be careful to stay away from health food store extracts or pills that claim to be made from green tea or similar plant extracts. There is no way to find out what other harmful additives these products may contain. You should always choose popular brand-name teas for consumption. If you have high blood pressure, heart disease, or diabetes, first check with your physician before trying green tea as a weight-reduction aid.

Tip 46 Go Ahead, Eat Chocolate!

Chocolate has long been the Achilles' heel of many dieters. Supposedly high in fat and calories, it has been considered a diet no-no for years. There is, however, some good news about chocolate that may cause you to rethink its value in a healthy diet. Besides tasting good, chocolate may have some healthy redeeming qualities.

Several recent studies indicate that chocolate is actually good for your heart. Dark chocolate is packed with antioxidant flavonoids, which can help to lower the bad LDL cholesterol, raise your good HDL cholesterol, and combat nasty free radicals that can cause cell damage. These antioxidants also help to prevent blood clots and inflammation in the arteries that supply blood to the heart. Studies have also shown that dark chocolate can reduce blood pressure in patients with high blood pressure.

Choose dark or bittersweet chocolate, which has three times as much flavonoids as milk chocolate. One study found that the cardioprotective effects of dark chocolate were reduced if the dark chocolate was consumed with milk (the combination then becomes milk chocolate, which appears to bind the antioxidants, making them unavailable for use in the body). Heating chocolate appears to release the antioxidants.

So if you're a chocolate lover, a good-tasting treat like chocolate won't hinder your diet program. A small chocolate-covered mint patty has only 1.5 grams of total fat and 0.8 grams of saturated fat. A small, thin square of dark chocolate has 3.5 grams of fat and 1.5 grams of saturated fat. Chocolate actually is good for weight loss, since it satisfies your sweet tooth and your brain's hunger mechanism, which prevents you from overeating. And chocolate also raises those good-feeling chemicals, endorphins, that help to relax and soothe the jangled nerves of the conscientious dieter. Enjoy!

PART 6

■

Diet Dos: Insider Secrets That Will Trim You Down

Tip 47 Diet One Day at a Time

Rome wasn't built in a day, and neither were you. It's easy to modify your eating habits by just taking small steps each week to change from poor eating habits to good ones. For long-term weight loss, make gradual changes to your lifestyle and diet. If you try to lose too much weight in too short a period of time, you're bound to get discouraged. Here are some good tips for dieting one day at a time:

- Don't concentrate on trying to lose fifteen pounds in the next month. Instead, set small, achievable weight-loss goals for yourself.
- Make gradual changes to your diet. For example, add more fruits to your diet one week and eat less high-calorie, high-fat foods the next week. The following week, add more vegetables to your meals and decrease the amount of starchy vegetables like corn and white potatoes. And the following week, substitute whole-grain cereals and breads for refined grains like white rice, white bread, and baked goods. Over time, you'll radically improve your diet without shocking your body or your taste buds by trying to do it all once.
- When you start an exercise program, don't try starting with two hours at the gym. Instead, make it your goal to walk fifteen minutes a day for the first two weeks. From there, increase to twenty minutes a day. From there, it's just a short jump to thirty minutes a day. Take walking breaks during lunch, after dinner, or in the morning, whenever it fits conveniently into your schedule. In no time, you'll start to feel healthier and more energetic, without going all out too fast.
- Before deciding to make changes to your diet, try just thinking about what you eat each day. Concentrate on eating your meals at regular intervals every day in the same place. Eat

only at the kitchen table, not in front of the TV, computer, or on the phone. Concentrate on eating slowly and only eating until you are no longer hungry, not until you are so full that you can't eat any more.

- Instead of trying to eliminate snacks from your diet, try adding healthier snacks to your diet. Opt for a piece of fruit or another low-fat, high-fiber option instead of a candy bar. This way you won't feel deprived, but you'll still be dieting.
- Dieting's no fun if you feel like you can't have something sweet once in a while. Instead of trying to radically eliminate dessert from your diet, come up with some desert options that make for lower fat, healthier alternatives to cake and ice cream. A nonfat yogurt will satisfy your sweet tooth at bedtime. Or treat yourself to a piece of dark chocolate.

Tip 48 Keep a Food and Exercise Diary

Oftentimes we underestimate how much we eat or lose track of how many desserts we cheat with each week. That's why it's a good idea to start a diet diary before you start any diet or exercise plan. In a small notebook, record the following:

1. The time you eat each meal.
2. What you ate and drank at each meal. Be specific, including amounts. Most important, be honest!
3. Include estimated portion sizes:
   • Your fist size is about ½ cup of pasta, rice, or vegetables.
   • Your palm size is about 3 to 4 ounces of protein.
4. Where were you when you ate? At home, at work, at a party?
5. Were you hungry?
6. Were you stressed, relaxed, bored, angry, or guilty?
7. Record physical activity for that day.
8. Weigh yourself once a week and record it.

After a week or two, look back over your entries to see what type of eater you are. This is a self-test, with no grades and no wrong answers:

1. Are you eating two, three, or four meals a day?
2. Do you snack regularly?
3. How long do you go between meals or snacks?
4. Are you eating because you are hungry or bored, angry, or guilty?
5. Do certain emotions trigger binge snack-food eating?

6. Are you eating healthy foods such as fruits, vegetables, lean protein, and whole-grain products?
7. Are you eating junk foods that are high in fat and calories?
8. How many calories are you eating daily, and how much fat and sugar do you consume?
9. Were you hungry when you ate, or did you just eat because you thought it was time to eat?
10. Are you getting any exercise at all?
11. Are you eating while watching TV or at the computer?
12. Do you eat late at night, just before bedtime?

Your diet diary is a necessary starting point to see what type of an eater and exerciser you are. After you've analyzed your self-test, you can start to adjust your eating and exercise habits in small steps accordingly.

Tip 49 Little Lifestyle Changes Make a Big Difference

Here's a list of helpful and easy lifestyle changes that go a long way toward helping you trim down.

- Eat more slowly with each meal. This involves taking smaller, less frequent bites and chewing each mouthful for a longer period of time. Pause between parts of the meal.
- If you are still hungry when you are finished with your first portion, wait at least fifteen minutes to see whether or not you really want another portion. In most cases, your appestat (the brain appetite control mechanism) will be more than satisfied at the end of that period of time, and you will not need a second helping.
- Keep foods out of sight between meals in your refrigerator or pantry. Do not leave food out where you can repeatedly see it during the day.
- Restrict your meals to one, or perhaps two, locations in your home for eating. If you have no regular place to eat, then you will find that you are eating in every room; however, when food is restricted to one main dining area, there will be fewer tendencies to snack during the day.
- Make it a point not to eat while watching television or reading, since you will eat more while not concentrating on your meal.
- Leave the table as soon as you are finished eating, and spend less time in the kitchen or areas that have a tendency to remind you of eating.

- Don't place serving dishes on the table during a meal, for there will be more of a tendency to take second and third helpings.
- Don't use food as a stress reliever. Most people have a tendency to seek out high-fat, high-sugar foods when under stress. Substitute music, exercise, meditation, or a warm bath for food cravings.
- Don't skip breakfast. People who do usually wind up having a high-fat, high-sugar snack such as a doughnut and coffee midmorning. A high-fiber, low-fat cereal with fruit and skim milk will hold you comfortably until lunchtime.
- Drink at least six 8-ounce glasses of water daily. Avoid drinking a lot of artificially sweetened drinks, as they will lower your blood sugar and thereby increase your appetite.
- Make your meals attractive with colorful foods, garnishes and greens, carrots, tomatoes, broccoli, spinach, peppers, yams, celery, and parsley in order to make them more appealing. Vary your meal plans daily to avoid boredom. Remember that the more colorful the foods are, the more phytonutrients they contain.
- Avoid sugar in sodas, teas, and fruit drinks. Use fresh orange juice, grapefruit juice, tomato juice (low sodium), and non-caffeinated teas, coffee, and diet sodas for snack drinks. Or make water (tap or bottled) your drink of choice.
- Avoid using cream, whole milk, or powdered creamers in your coffee or tea. Substitute skim milk. Nondairy creamers may contain trans fats. Check for the words "hydrogenated" or "partially hydrogenated" on ingredient labels.
- Choose skim milk. It has no fat, has all of the calcium, vitamins, and minerals that are present in 1 percent, 2 percent, or whole milk, and it tastes just as good.
- Don't start a weight-reduction program just prior to the holiday season or before a vacation, since these are the most unsuccessful times to begin this type of project.

- Eat salad greens and vegetables before the main course, since these will take the edge off your hunger for higher-calorie meat, poultry, and fish portions.
- The best salad dressing is none. Salad dressings are high in fats and calories. Use calorie-free herbs, spices, lemon, vinegar, or occasionally a small amount of nonfat or low-fat, low-calorie dressing. If you must have the full-fat version, dip your fork in a side cup of salad dressing every few mouthfuls of salad and you'll enjoy the taste without the extra calories.
- Fresh or frozen vegetables and fruits are better choices than canned fruits and vegetables, which can be loaded with salt or sugar.
- Hot foods, such as soups, and foods that require a lot of chewing will leave you with a greater feeling of satisfaction because they take a longer time to swallow and absorb.
- Always trim away visible fat from meat and poultry before cooking, and remove visible fat at the table when eating. Canned fishes, such as tuna and salmon, should be packed in water or have the oils drained away.
- Teflon-coated pans and the new nonfat edible spray-on coatings, which are made of vegetable oil, will help reduce the amount of caloric fat that you consume.
- Don't go grocery shopping when you're hungry or you'll wind up buying impulse, high-fat snack foods. Prepare a list of healthy items before you go and don't deviate from it.
- When shopping for packaged or canned goods, make sure the item of food you are purchasing has no more than 1.5 to 2.0 grams of saturated fat per serving. If it is higher, look for another brand. Always look for nonfat or low-fat products; however, remember to look at the nutrition facts information, and don't depend on a label that says "low-fat food." Many so-called low-fat items are fairly high in total fat content; for example, 2 percent milk has 5 grams of fat, or 98 percent fat-free yogurt can have 3.5 to 4.0 grams of total fat. Always

choose foods that contain no more than 2.0 grams of saturated fat.

- Excessive alcohol is one of the most serious hazards in any diet program, whether you are dining out or at home. The additional calories consumed in the American diet from alcohol have a tendency to cause and maintain overweight. Alcohol has more calories than most foods (7 calories per gram). Try to substitute club soda with a twist of lemon, or mineral water, for drinks. Limit your alcohol intake to 4 ounces of red wine or 12 ounces of light beer three times per week.

Tip 50 Calculte Your BMI Goal

The Body Mass Index, commonly known as the BMI, is the new measurement to indicate if you are obese or just considered overweight. The BMI is a relatively complicated formula based on your weight in pounds and your height in inches. It's much easier to consult BMI tables in health magazine or web sites.

The BMI uses a mathematical formula that takes into account both a person's height and weight. BMI equals a person's weight in kilograms divided by height in meters squared.

$$BMI = \frac{kg}{(m)^2}$$

An easier method of calculating the BMI is to divide your weight (in pounds) by the square of your height (in inches) and then multiply by 703. For example, if you weigh 150 pounds and are 5′5″ (65 inches) you would:

1. Multiply 65 by 65 to determine height squared = 4225
2. Divide 150 (pounds) by 4225 (height squared) = 0.036
3. Multiply 0.036 by 703 = 25 (which is your BMI)

BODY MASS INDEX

BMI	Weight	Heart Disease Risk
18.5–24.9	Normal	None
25.0–29.9	Overweight	Increased
30.0–34.9	Obese	High
35.0–39.9	Obese	Very High
40.0 or greater	Extremely Obese	Extremely High

Heart disease and strokes are the leading causes of disability and death in the United States, and being overweight increases your risk of developing either or both of these diseases. People who are over-weight are also twice as likely to develop adult-onset diabetes.

But if you aren't at your target weight right now, don't panic! By just increasing physical activity to thirty minutes of walking every other day and losing 5 to 10 percent of your current weight, you decrease the risk of heart disease, strokes, and diabetes by more than 50 percent. Studies have shown that overweight or obese people who exercise regularly and modify their diets have improvements in blood pressure, diabetic control, heart function, blood fats (choles-terol and triglycerides), sleep disorders, and, in general, have improved feelings of well-being and self-esteem.

By calculating your diet goal, you've already taken the first step toward a healthier you.

Tip 51 Beat Food Cravings with These Tips

Food cravings may have a physiological as well as an emotional component, according to many researchers. Those cravings for ice cream, pizza, and hoagies may not necessarily begin in the stomach. Here are some ideas on how to tackle diet-sabotaging cravings.

Physical Food Cravings

Sometimes your cravings are physical. Here are some ways to deal with them:

Carbohydrate Cravings

That craving you have for carbs like sweets, cakes, pretzels, potato chips, and crackers may be caused by low blood sugar. This condition can occur when you have not eaten for several hours or because of emotional frustration, and has been noted to be present prior to women's menstrual period because of hormonal fluctuations. Complex carbohydrates such as fruits, vegetables, and whole-grain cereals can reduce the craving for refined carbohydrates. High-protein, nonfat milk and low-fat or skim milk cheese can also cut this craving.

Salt Cravings

Your yearning for salty foods such as pickles, potato chips, and olives, can result from salt depletion caused by excessive perspiration or from a stress condition that results in stimulation of the adrenal glands. Salt cravings can be reduced by substituting lemon juice and herbs. Adding fresh fruit that has a high vitamin C content (orange, grapefruit, banana, cantaloupe, tomato, or strawberries) to the diet can reduce the craving for salt.

Caffeine

Caffeine is a stimulant that is present in coffee, tea, and cola drinks. Cocoa and chocolate contain theobromine, a caffeine-type substance. Many people are actually addicted both physiologically and metabolically to caffeine and will suffer withdrawal symptoms, which include headache, fatigue, nausea, and irritability, as well as a craving for sugar. To reduce this addiction, you have to gradually reduce the caffeine in your diet by substituting noncaffeinated drinks such as decaffeinated coffee, herbal teas, clear diet sodas other than colas, and mineral water or club soda.

Emotions and Food Cravings

Emotions definitely play a role in food cravings. Here are some of the most common craving-causing emotions and what you can do to overcome them before they overcome your good diet intentions:

Anxiety and Stress

People who are anxious or stressed out have a tendency to crave sweets and high-calorie foods. Anxiety and stress cause your adrenal glands and pituitary gland to produce certain hormones that stimulate your brain's hunger mechanism to crave refined sugars and carbohydrates (cakes, pies, doughnuts, and candy bars). These quick-fix carbs tend to quell anxiety temporarily by the sudden rise in blood sugar, which causes a feeling of calm. However, with the rapid rise in blood sugar comes a rapid spike in insulin and a more rapid drop in blood sugar, causing anxiety to quickly return.

You can beat food cravings caused by anxiety and stress by eating low-calorie, crunchy foods such as apples, celery, carrot sticks, or low-fat whole wheat or sourdough pretzels. The crunch factor gives your stress-induced anxiety time to cool down without causing a rapid rise in your blood sugar. The process of chewing also causes your facial and neck muscles to relax, which relieves stress and tension.

Depression and Sadness

If you are depressed or sad, your first inclination may be to head for the sweet bar instead of the salad bar. The quick fix of sugar raises the blood sugar, which in turn spikes the pancreas's insulin production. High levels of insulin in the blood increase the production of serotonin, which improves your mood. You feel more relaxed and mellow, which is actually how antidepressant drugs work, by increasing your brain's serotonin levels.

Unfortunately, serotonin levels plummet after insulin levels drop, and the feelings of sadness and depression quickly return. To combat this feeling, you can boost your serotonin levels for longer periods of time by eating fruits when you are feeling down. Fruits only gradually increase the level of blood sugar because fruit sugar, or fructose, is absorbed slowly. Insulin levels then become graduated, causing a sustained, long-lived increase in blood and brain serotonin levels.

Boredom

People who eat because they are bored or just plain tired often eat high-calorie refined sugar carbohydrate snacks like cakes and candies, which are readily available and easy to buy and consume. A caffeinated mocha latte may taste good, but the caffeine and sugar interfere with the production of endorphins and serotonin. Instead of feeling relaxed and calm afterward, you will feel edgy and wired.

Nuts, particularly almonds and walnuts, are great boredom snacks, since they provide omega-3 fatty acids that can relieve the feelings of fatigue and boredom. Combined with raisins, nuts make the ideal feel-good, energy-boosting snack.

Discontent

People who are unhappy or in a bad mood often turn to high-fat, high-carbohydrate foods like pizza or cheese steaks smothered in onions. These foods contain protein and fat, both of which help to produce good-feeling endorphins. They also have tons of fat and calories, which help to destroy any well-intentioned diet plan.

To increase your endorphins without packing on pounds, substitute high-fiber, whole-grain cereals and breads for refined carbs and substitute lean protein, low-fat cheeses, yogurt, turkey, chicken, and fish for the unwanted extra fat calories. These complex carbohydrates and high-protein foods produce both endorphins and serotonin to keep your mood happy and euphoric, so you boost your mood with less fat and less calories.

Tip 52 Try This Simple 20/20 Weight-Loss Formula

To meet your target weight loss, try this easy 20/20 formula: eat no more than 20 grams of total fat calories daily, and eat at least 20 grams of dietary fiber daily.

Eat Less than 20 Grams of Total Fat a Day

Excess fat in the diet causes heart disease, diabetes, cardiovascular disease, and breast and uterine cancer. Less fat in the diet results in more stored fat being burned as fuel so both you and your fat cells become nice and thin.

- Fat contains 9 calories per gram, whereas both carbohydrate and protein contain only 4 calories per gram. (One pound of body fat contains 3,500 calories.)
- Fat is the number one killer of both your heart and your figure.
- Consult a chart for the total grams of fat in various foods and keep a record of what you eat.
- To maintain your ideal weight, eat no more than 20 grams of fat daily.

Eat at Least 20 Grams of Dietary Fiber Daily

- Fiber helps you lose weight because eating fiber-rich foods leads to slower emptying of the stomach that makes you feel full earlier. Fiber contains fewer calories for its large volume (called a high bulk ratio) so that it satisfies your hunger center more quickly and fills you up without filling you out. It has the ability to absorb lots of water and therefore regulates the progression of food through the digestive system. Fiber helps to lower blood cholesterol and also decreases the risk of heart disease, hypertension, and stroke.

- Fruits, vegetables, and whole grains are not only high in fiber but also contain many nutrients and antioxidants.
- Consult a chart for the total grams of fiber in various foods and keep a record of what you eat.
- To maintain your ideal weight, eat no less than 20 grams of dietary fiber daily.

Tip 53 Dine in More Often

The increase in obesity coincides with the increased number of meals eaten out at restaurants. With our busy, on-the-go lifestyles, more and more we wind up eating out or getting our meals from takeout or fast-food restaurants. This poses a lot of dieting problems. For one, restaurants usually serve huge portions, portions that are far larger than what you might make for yourself at home. Moreover, while you can make healthful choices in your own kitchen, you don't have as much say over how your restaurant meal is prepared.

The best solution for this is to make a concentrated effort to eat more meals at home. See Part 8, "Try These Meals and Fat-Melting Tips in the Kitchen and On the Go," for some healthy meal options. If you know you'll be at the office all day but are trying to watch what you eat, pack yourself a low-fat lunch the night before with a couple of healthy snacks to tide you over. If your schedule doesn't allow you to cook every night, try making two or three meals on days when you do have time, like weekends, and then having healthy leftovers during the week.

And when you must eat out, don't finish those oversized meals that most restaurants put in front of you. Eat half the meal and take the other half home, or share with a friend or family member. Check out Tip 79, "Tips for Eating Well While Eating Out," to help you make smart choices.

Tip 54 Walk Before and After Eating

Studies show that walking before meals decreases your appetite. (See Tip 85.) In addition, walking approximately forty-five minutes to an hour after eating increases the body's metabolic rate to burn away calories at a faster rate.

This burning of calories at a faster rate has been explained as a combination of the energy expended from walking and the calories burned in the digestion of food itself. (See Tip 90.) We actually burn more calories after we eat because the energy metabolism of the body increases 5 to 10 percent. This doesn't mean that the more you eat, the more calories you'll burn. But it is a good reason for walking forty-five minutes to an hour after small meals for additional weight loss.

The combination of walking before and after meals will help you take in fewer calories and burn off more so you lose weight faster and more easily. See Part 9, "Get Moving," for more information on the benefits of exercise and how to start a walking and exercise program.

Tip 55 Trim Your Tummy with These Fat-Busting Tips

We all have our own weight-loss problem zone, the place we'd really like to trim down. Unsightly belly fat is one of the most common problem areas. Here are some tips that will target your tummy and help you trim down.

Avoid Saturated Fats

People whose diets are high in saturated fats are prone to storing fat in the abdomen, surrounding vital organs such as the liver, pancreas, and intestinal tract. This type of fat is referred to as visceral fat and puts these individuals at risk for developing diabetes, fatty liver, and heart disease. This abdominal or *visceral fat* is the direct result of eating saturated fats such as fatty meats, deli meats, cheeses, butter, whole milk products, and prepackaged foods made with hydrogenated or partially hydrogenated oils that contain the bad trans fats.

Unfortunately, in some cases, genetics plays a role in developing excess abdominal fat. In these cases you should make an extra effort to limit saturated fat products to no more than 10 percent of your total daily calorie intake. In those individuals who have the genetic trait for developing excessive abdominal fat and also have high levels of blood fats no matter how hard they try to diet, a physician should be consulted regarding the possibility of taking a cholesterol lowering medication.

Avoid Refined Carbs

The refined carbohydrates we eat are quickly absorbed into the bloodstream, which causes a sudden spike in insulin production.

This excess amount of insulin causes the digested refined carbohydrates to head straight into our fat cells. Because the fat cells in the belly are located close to the digestive tract and because the abdomen contains the most concentrated number of fat cells in the body, most of the fat from refined carbohydrates heads straight to the belly. Once the excess insulin has done its work of dropping the blood sugar and packing fat into your belly fat cells, it results in low blood sugar that causes another round of carbohydrate cravings. It's a lose-lose combination.

As we age, we crave more carbohydrates, and the more carbs we eat, the more calories are stored as fat in our abdomens. Due to certain hormonal changes that regulate our digestive system, we become less able to burn carbs as fuel, thus making carbs more likely to be stored as fat. This becomes a vicious cycle, because the carbs we store as belly fat actually cause an increase in our craving for more carbohydrates. Stored abdominal fat suppresses the formation of a fat-burning hormone called *leptin*, which helps to keep blood sugar steady. Consequently, the more abdominal fat you store, the easier it becomes to gain more weight, because less leptin is being produced and subsequently less fat is being burned.

If you avoid saturated fats and refined carbs, you will begin to lose abdominal fat. If you can lose abdominal fat, then you will diminish carbohydrate cravings, and subsequently lose more unwanted belly fat.

■ White Bread and Abdominal Fat

According to a new study from Tufts University in Boston, people who eat too much white bread have larger waistlines than those individuals who eat whole grains. White bread appears to go straight to the abdomen to be stored as belly fat. People who ate the most white bread were also the fattest and had a higher risk of heart disease compared to those who didn't carry the extra weight around the belly.

Eat High-Fiber Foods

By eating high-fiber foods, you can actually block the absorption of refined carbohydrates and starches by forming a web or network of fibers that encircles these starches. This fiber web carries the starches out of the digestive tract almost completely intact and undigested. By blocking most of the absorption of these refined starches, less sugar and insulin are present in the bloodstream, which results in less craving for carbohydrates. The less you crave carbs, the more belly fat you burn and the more weight you lose, particularly around the abdomen.

Some high-fiber foods, particularly beans (white, kidney, fava, chick peas), contain an enzyme-blocking compound that blocks the pancreatic enzymes amylase and lipase from breaking down refined starches. Because these pancreatic enzymes are inhibited from absorbing refined carbohydrates, your digestive tract bypasses the absorption of these starches and they are transported out of the body. This results in a much slower rise in blood sugar, which in turn doesn't cause a spike in insulin production and consequently reduces your craving for carbohydrates. This results in less fat stored in your belly.

Walk It Off

Even though there is no magic diet for getting rid of abdominal fat, eating the proper foods and walking helps get rid of it. An aerobic exercise such as walking is the secret formula that can strengthen your abdominal muscles and help you to lose abdominal fat.

First of all, when you walk briskly with an even stride, you are contracting and relaxing muscles in your chest, back, and abdomen. With each forward motion of your legs, these muscles contract to keep your body erect. Your abdominal muscles tighten automatically, exactly as they would if you were doing strenuous sit-ups, with one exception—you're not straining your back! As you walk, your upper body chest wall muscles aid in tightening the lower abdominal muscles. This combination of upper body and lower abdominal muscle contractions is what produces a firm, flat tummy.

Walking regularly tightens abdominal muscles and helps to burn away belly fat, and as an added bonus it will also help to trim down your hips, thighs, and buttocks. Since walking is a moderate aerobic exercise, it burns fat rather than carbohydrates. When this walking fat-burning exercise is combined with light handheld weights (see Tip 96), you can speed up the abdominal flattening process as you burn fat and build muscle.

And remember that often the last place that you've gained weight is the first place the weight will come off when you cut the saturated fat out of your diet. So if you have started to gain abdominal fat, you may notice that you'll lose inches around your middle when you start your low-fat diet. When you reduce your fat and calorie intake, you will lose weight all over your body, including that unsightly belly fat.

Tip 56 Eat Like the French!

Nutritionists, doctors, and dieters have all been touting the French diet—and for good reason. The French have only had an 8 to 10 percent rise in obesity over the last decade, compared to a 20 to 25 percent increase in obesity in the American population. Also, the French have considerably less heart disease and breast cancer compared to Americans. So pass on the all-American burgers and fries and try these healthy French diet tricks; your body—and waist-line—will thank you.

The French Paradox

While people in France eat almost twice as much saturated fat as Americans, the French have only one-third the risk of heart disease. They owe their heart health in part to *le vin rouge*, or red wine.

There are three known factors that contribute to atherosclerosis, or hardening of the arteries:

- Excessive platelet activity, which causes blood cells to stick together and can lead to a heart attack or stroke.
- High levels of bad LDL cholesterol. Free radicals can oxidize LDL cholesterol and contribute to the buildup of plaque in the arteries.
- Damage to endothelial cells that line the heart and blood vessels.

A diet high in purple grapes has been found to cause an increase in the flexibility of the body's blood vessels. When blood vessels have increased flexibility they dilate or widen and blood can flow more easily through them to all of the body's cells, tissues, and organs. This increase in blood flow also helps to slow the oxidation of LDL (bad cholesterol), thus decreasing the chance of cholesterol being deposited in the arteries (atherosclerosis or the hardening of the arteries). The key to the prevention of atherosclerosis is the flavonoid called transresveratrol, which is present in purple grapes. The same heart disease prevention benefits appear to be related to the consumption of red wine, which contains the same flavonoids as purple grapes (*Circulation* 100: 1050–1055; October 1999), which increases the good HDL cholesterol.

This research is often referred to as the French paradox, and helps to explain the low incidence of heart disease in France, where red wine consumption is high. Eating purple grapes or grape juice gives similar protection against heart disease without the alcohol content as both contain flavonoids with cardioprotective benefits.

Bon Appetit!

It is not only the wine that keeps the French people healthy, however, it's their preparation and enjoyment of healthy, fresh foods and their relaxed manner of eating slow, leisurely meals. The French take time preparing and eating their meals, unlike their American counterparts, who eat fast food and prepare fast meals and eat them just as fast, without paying attention to how much they are actually eating. Try savoring foods like the French do and taking the same care in food preparation and presentation.

The French also eat three to four more servings of vegetables daily than Americans eat, and they season their vegetables with heart-friendly olive oil, fresh herbs, nuts, and spices. They usually sauté or grill their fresh vegetables to bring out the natural sugars and nutrients contained in the vegetables. In contrast to whopping American portions, the French eat relatively small portions of meat in comparison to the amount of fresh vegetables they consume. Plus, French people rarely eat prepackaged foods, which are filled with saturated fats, sugar, and sodium. And even though they enjoy desserts with a high fat content, they usually only consume small portions.

Tip 57 Dine the Mediterranean Way

Mediterranean cultures have been thriving on a nutritious diet of whole grains, olive oil, vegetables, legumes, nuts, seeds, potatoes, fruits, and fish, with very little meat and whole-fat dairy products, for thousands of years. Research shows that the Mediterranean diet is far healthier then the typical American diet, which is high in fat and processed foods. Mediterranean cultures have a significantly decreased risk of heart disease and cancer—an approximately 35 percent reduced risk of mortality due to coronary heart disease and a 25 percent reduced risk of mortality due to cancer.

The Health Benefits

A twelve-year study published in the September 2004 issue of the *Journal of the American Medical Association* reported that the mortality rates were 65 percent lower in elderly people who followed the Mediterranean diet and who walked thirty minutes daily. Researchers also found that the Mediterranean diet contributed to a significant decrease in body weight, blood pressure, cholesterol and triglycerides, and blood sugar and insulin levels. At the same time, the Mediterranean diet significantly increases the good HDL cholesterol, which helps to prevent heart disease. This twelve-year study followed approximately twenty-five hundred men and women ages seventy to ninety in eleven European countries.

A separate study also reported in the September 2004 issue of the *Journal of the American Medical Association* found that the Mediterranean diet helped people lose weight by actually changing their body chemistry, reducing dangerous insulin abnormalities and decreasing chronic inflammation of arteries and other tissues in the body. This diet reduced the incidence of this metabolic syndrome, which causes the accumulation of fat around the abdomen and increases the risk of diabetes, heart disease, cancer, and Alzheimer's disease.

How to Eat the Mediterranean Way

Many of the Mediterranean diet's health benefits are due to its emphasis on whole grains. Grains consist of three layers: the inner germ, the middle endosperm, and the outer bran. Processing white flour and white rice keeps the two inside layers but removes the outside layer, the bran, with its fiber, vitamins, and minerals. With whole grains, you get all of those nutrients plus complex carbohydrates, protein, fiber, antioxidants, and other phytochemicals that may help guard against cancer and heart disease.

Also, whole grains provide energy and calories with little fat and are digested more slowly so that you feel full longer. The Mediterranean diet is far superior to the traditional Western diet because fiber is a significantly important factor in weight reduction and good health. Weight control is aided by the slower emptying of the stomach when you ingest soluble fiber. This also causes a feeling of fullness and a decrease in hunger, causing fewer calories to be consumed.

In addition to whole grains, the Mediterranean diet is rich in olive oil, vegetables, legumes, fish, chicken, fruits, and pasta and light on red meat. Although their diet contains 25 to 35 percent fat calories, this fat is monounsaturated, heart-healthy fat. Mediterraneans use olive oil and olives in almost everything they eat, including pastas, breads, vegetables, salads, fish, and even in cakes and pastries. Olive oil's monounsaturated fats help to increase the good HDL cholesterol and decrease the bad LDL cholesterol. This leads to less cholesterol blocking the arteries and a significantly lower incidence of heart attacks and strokes. Olive oil also contains certain antioxidants called polyphenols, which have cancer-protective qualities.

And if all that isn't enough to help the Mediterraneans keep healthy, they also have a secret weapon: walking! To complement their healthy diet, Mediterraneans walk almost all of the time. They walk to work, to visit friends, or just to leisurely stroll through their cities and countrysides. They climb up and down hills and keep in good shape with little or no thought to their aerobic activity.

Tip 58 Eat Smaller, More Frequent Meals

Have you ever noticed thin, wiry people who seem to be eating all the time, but never get fat? That's because they eat small, frequent meals that are lower in calories, and their metabolism seems to burn them up at a faster rate, rather than having to deal with a large number of calories all at once.

After a meal, the pancreas (an endocrine gland located behind your stomach) produces a hormone called insulin, which is released into the bloodstream. A meal that is high in fat or sugar causes the pancreas to release a lot more insulin than does a meal high in complex carbohydrates. Likewise, a larger meal causes more insulin to be released than a smaller meal. One of insulin's functions is to regulate the level of sugar in the blood by burning carbohydrates and conserving stores of body fat in the body's fat cells, where it can later be burned as fuel for energy. High levels of insulin promote the absorption of dietary fat into the body's fat cells. In other words, the amount of fat in the cells increases as the insulin levels become higher. In addition, less fat can be released from the body's fat cells while insulin levels remain elevated.

More frequent, smaller meals, on the other hand, tend to keep the pancreas from producing excess amounts of insulin. This results in more dietary fat being burned as fuel, which results in less fat being stored in the fat cells. Also, a lower insulin level encourages the breakdown of fat already in your fat cells to be released into the blood and used as an additional fuel for energy.

In other words, eating small, frequent complex carbohydrate meals leads to steadier, lower levels of insulin being released into the bloodstream than does eating larger, high-fat, high-sugar meals; therefore smaller, frequent complex carbohydrate meals result in more fat being burned as a fuel and less fat being stored as fat deposits. This is because as you burn more fat, you are actually using up calories instead of storing calories. As an added benefit of eating small, frequent complex carbohydrate meals, you actually will notice a decrease in your appetite. The reason your appetite is decreased is twofold. First, because your blood sugar doesn't get too low, you do not experience hunger pangs. Second, the fact that complex carbo-hydrates take longer to digest also causes a decrease in hunger. This is because your appetite-control mechanism (appestat), signals to you that you are full. Complex carbohydrates stay in the stomach and intestines longer because they are absorbed at a much slower rate than refined sugars and carbohydrates.

PART 7

■

Diet Don'ts: Don't Let These Diet Traps Trip You Up

Tip 59 Don't Panic If You Plateau

Remember, no one loses weight in a straight line. When you are on a diet, you initially lose weight, and then your weight loss levels off. This occurs even though you are eating exactly the same amount as you were when you lost the initial weight. This leveling-off period or *plateau* is the single most hazardous part of any diet program because once this plateau is reached, you begin to become discouraged and say, "I'm still on the same diet, but I haven't lost a pound in over a week." Discouragement leads to frustration, and next you'll say, "The heck with the diet. I may as well enjoy myself and eat something I really like, since I haven't lost weight anyway." At this point, 90 percent of all diets are doomed to failure, since the weight-loss pattern now reverses itself and becomes a weight-gain pattern.

The thing to remember is that this plateau period is always temporary. If you can stick it out, you'll be surprised to see that the weight loss begins to pick up speed again. It may take a week or two, at the most, but if you are patient, you will again start to lose those unwanted pounds. No one has ever satisfactorily explained this plateau period; however, physiologists believe that it is probably due to a temporary readjustment of the body's metabolism in response to the initial weight loss. No matter what the reason is, however, you will always break through the plateau period, providing you don't become discouraged or frustrated. Weight loss will again resume its downward progress toward your goal.

Tip 60 Don't Weigh Yourself Every Day

Weighing yourself every day is hazardous to your diet. The reason for this is twofold. First, when you weigh yourself daily and see that you are losing weight, you become happy and elated, and subconsciously you will eat to celebrate. Second, if you see that you are not losing weight as fast as you think you should, you become depressed and anxious, and sometime during that day you will subconsciously eat because of frustration. So the rule of thumb is, the more you weigh yourself, the more you eat!

Believe me, it is true. I've seen my patients go through this frustrating daily weighing process thousands of times. If you are dieting you should not weigh yourself more than once a week, and then you will get a true measure of the effectiveness of your diet. If you must weigh yourself, Wednesday is the best day to weigh yourself each week. Monday and Friday are the worst days for weighing in because they follow and precede the weekend and can lead to frustrating eating binges. It took a long time to gain all that weight; you can't take it off overnight. Be patient!

Tip 61 Don't Skip Meals

You may think that skipping breakfast or lunch would be a good way to cut calories—it's not! Skipping meals lowers your blood sugar, which brings on cravings for high-carbohydrate, high-calorie foods. It is far better for you and your diet to eat three to four, even five small meals a day than one or two large meals, because the smaller meals throughout the day will keep your blood sugar on an even keel. If your blood sugar remains constant, you are less likely to overeat and gain weight.

Similarly, fasting does not lead to weight loss, because when you fast your body thinks you are starving and attempts to conserve calories by slowing your body metabolism considerably. Because you burn calories at a much slower rate it's unlikely you will lose any weight at all by fasting. Besides, once you resume your food intake, your body's metabolism remains in its slowed-down phase until it's sure you're not starving. During this time, most of the calories you eat get stored in fat cells, and you are likely to gain extra weight instead of losing weight.

Start Your Day Off Right

People who never eat breakfast usually make up for it sometime during the day, and then some. By the time lunch comes, your low blood sugar gives you a ravenous appetite and you're sure to overeat. Or you may get hungry long before lunchtime arrives, and you'll end up devouring doughnuts and coffee. People who skip breakfast seem to make up for it threefold by snacking midmorning, midafternoon, and late evening.

When you skip breakfast, your body thinks you are starving, and in response it slows your metabolism. This results in sluggishness and fatigue, which in turn cause you to "just eat something" in order to feel better. Eating speeds up the metabolism and elevates the blood sugar, and lo and behold, you feel better. Then the blood sugar rapidly drops again, and you feel fatigued again, and so you eat again. This is called *functional hypoglycemia* or low blood sugar, which results from just skipping meals.

▓ The Most Successful Dieters Eat Breakfast

Studies show that people who eat a healthy breakfast every day are the most successful dieters. Healthy breakfasts of whole-grain, high-fiber cereal topped with fruit and skim milk are a great way to start the day, or an egg fried in a small amount of olive oil on a slice of toasted whole wheat bread makes a great lean protein meal. A slice of whole wheat bread topped with a tablespoon of all-fruit jelly and/or natural peanut butter is an appetite-satisfying breakfast. People who regularly eat a healthy breakfast don't get hungry for midmorning snacks of doughnuts or muffins. Your body's appetite control mechanism stays in check for long periods of time, without any spikes in blood sugar or blood insulin levels. And besides, a nutritious breakfast causes your body to burn fat more efficiently and starts your day off perfectly.

Tip 62   Don't Let Peer Pressure Pile on the Pounds

Research shows that people eat more when they are dining with more people. With the excitement of dining with friends, your appetite goes into overdrive and your appetite mechanism doesn't shut off easily, since you're talking and having fun. Before you know it, you're eating much more than you should have eaten, without realizing the total amount of food you have consumed. This is especially true if the people you are eating with consume larger amounts of food.

Plan in advance if you're going to have dinner with friends. Order a low-fat, low-calorie meal, regardless of what your dinner companions order. If you're a woman dining with a man, you should know that, in general, men can eat much more food than women can without gaining weight. Who said life was fair! Men burn more calories quickly because of testosterone that builds muscle mass, which causes their metabolism to run faster.

Here are some tips to help you eat less when you're dining with friends or family:

- Chew your food slowly.
- Put your fork down between bites.
- Stop eating when talking and resume eating slowly when conversation stops.
- Don't be afraid to leave food on your plate.
- If you're eating at home, when you feel full take your plate into the kitchen and return to the table. If there is no plate, there is no more food to pick at.
- Never order a meal to coincide with what your friends are ordering. Fatty, high-calorie meals sound good when some-

one else orders them; however, don't let their order be contagious. One way to avoid temptation is to order your meal first.

- Don't try to keep up the pace with a fast eater at your table. This person probably has no idea what or how much he or she is eating. Fast eaters are usually talking a mile a minute while eating nonstop.
- Be careful of alcoholic beverages when dining with friends. Never order more than one drink. If you're not a drinker, don't be afraid to not order a drink. Just get water or club soda with a twist. If you'd like a light drink, however, get a white wine spritzer (half the wine, half the calories, and club soda).
- Don't feel pressured to finish your entire plate. The portions at restaurants are two to three times as large as they would be at home. It might be helpful to have the waiter package half the meal to go before you even begin to eat.

Tip 63 Don't Deprive Yourself of Your Favorite Foods

It isn't what you eat that makes you fat, it's how much you eat or how many calories you consume. So it's really not necessary to severely restrict your diet and deny yourself your favorite foods. If you just eat less of the so-called forbidden foods, you'll satisfy your cravings without sabotaging your diet, and you won't be tempted to binge on those forbidden favorites.

If You Have a Weakness for Pasta, Potatoes, and Bread

Bad carbs are certainly tempting. Whenever possible, try to satisfy your carbohydrate craving healthfully by eating whole-grain varieties of your favorite carbs. If you're craving a potato, eat it with the skin or have a good-carb sweet potato instead.

Be sure to eat protein along with any bad carbs you crave. The protein will decrease your craving for additional bad carbs. Plus protein is more filling than carbs, so you'll eat fewer calories with a protein-carb meal than you would if you just consumed the refined carbohydrates alone. Protein takes longer to digest and fills you up faster, while providing few calories and increased nutrition.

Research has shown that adding protein to each meal produces a higher body temperature and, therefore, a higher basal metabolic rate. This increases the number of calories burned in any twenty-four-hour period. Protein-enriched meals take considerably longer to digest than carbohydrate meals and therefore not only make you feel full earlier, but also contribute to a prolonged burning of calories, particularly stored fat, resulting in more weight loss.

The best protein foods to add to bad-carb meals include lean meat and poultry, fish; peanut butter; nuts; legumes; low-fat or nonfat milk, yogurt, and cheese; hard-boiled eggs; soy products; and sunflower or sesame seeds. The worst proteins include marbled meats, hamburgers and cheeseburgers, high-fat dairy products, and processed meats. Bacon, sausage, and Canadian bacon are bad; however, a slice of extra-lean ham has only 1 gram of fat and 38 calories.

When You Have a Sweet Tooth for Cookies, Cakes, Ice Cream, or Candy

Try to outsmart your cravings before they start by keeping portable food handy whenever you go out. If you munch on an apple, orange, banana, or pear when your sweet tooth surfaces, you'll take in fewer calories and more fiber ounce for ounce from these healthy sweets.

If your appetite, however, goes into overdrive, and you must have a forbidden sweet, then have it. Take one or two bites of the sweet and chew slowly; throw the rest of it away or share it with a dining companion. Your sweet tooth will be satisfied, and you won't take in the extra fat and calories.

The best sweets to have are fruits, nonfat dessert gelatin or pudding with nonfat whipped topping, lightly sugared whole-grain cereal bites, a small amount of nonfat or low-fat ice cream, low-fat or nonfat yogurt, a slice of angel food cake with a tablespoon of nonfat fudge, or a smoothie of nonfat milk or yogurt blended with your favorite fruit. Diet soft drinks can also satisfy your sweet tooth. The worst sweets are cakes, candy bars, regular sodas, cookies, doughnuts, pastries, candies, and fruit juices.

When You Must Have Something Fattening

Let's face it—fat adds flavor to food and makes it taste good. When you're craving high-fat foods, concentrate on eating the good fats, which actually taste as good as the bad fats:

- Instead of a cup of tuna salad with full-fat mayonnaise (20 grams of fat and 400 calories), use a small can of water-packed tuna with nonfat mayo (3 grams of fat and 225 calories) for your sandwich or salad.
- Instead of bacon or sausage with your eggs, choose low-fat, lean ham (1 slice), which only has 1 gram of fat and 40 calories.
- Instead of full-fat cream cheese on your bagel (scooped out), use nonfat cream cheese and you'll save lots of fat and calories.
- Low-fat or nonfat cottage cheese tastes as good as the whole-fat variety, with a lot less calories and fat.
- Substitute low-fat or nonfat salad dressings or olive oil instead of full-fat salad dressings for your salads. Or better yet, use lemon juice or flavored vinegars, which have no calories at all.
- Substitute 2 egg whites for each whole egg, and you'll save 80 calories and 10 grams of fat.
- Instead of full-fat potato chips, make your own potato chips by slicing a small potato into thin slices and baking in the oven with olive oil vegetable spray. Add herbs if you'd like to vary the taste.
- Substitute low-fat ice cream or low-fat yogurt instead of the whole-milk, whole-fat variety. The minimal fat content present in the low-fat yogurt and ice cream tastes just as good as the whole-fat variety.

• Lean turkey or breast of chicken makes a nutritious, lean protein sandwich on whole wheat bread with nonfat mayo.

Keep in mind which fats are healthier for you than others. The best fats for you to eat come from nuts, legumes, peanut butter, avocado, and canola and olive oils. The worst fats come from breaded or fried foods; cream soups and sauces; whole-fat mayo and salad dressings; processed foods such as crackers, cookies, and chips with trans fats; marbled meats; and butter, margarine, and cooking oils, except for olive and canola oils.

Tip 64 Don't Believe the Cellulite Myth

They are all over: the special creams, diets, and exercises that are meant to target the nastiest of all nasty fats—cellulite. Well, whatever they are selling, don't buy it, because cellulite is actually a myth. In the end, it's no different than any other fat cell, and it doesn't require any special treatments to get rid of it. When fat cells immediately beneath the skin enlarge, sometimes the strands of fibrous tissue that connect these fat cells don't stretch. This gives ordinary fat a lumpy appearance on the hips, thighs, and buttocks, which has been given the mythical name *cellulite* by gimmick diet promoters.

In a recent study conducted at Johns Hopkins University in Baltimore, fat biopsies were taken from people with lumpy fatty tissues (the mythical cellulite) and from people with regular fat deposits. The result: all of the biopsy specimens were identified under the microscope as ordinary fat cells. There was no tissue identified as cellulite!

So don't be fooled by the cellulite myth and buy any special cellulite treatments. And don't be discouraged if you notice that the fat on your hips, thighs or buttocks has a lumpier appearance than elsewhere. The truth is that cellulite is ordinary fat that you can fight through ordinary means. A low-fat diet combined with a regular aerobic walking program will melt away fat wherever it is located on your body.

Tip 65 Don't Fall for These Diet Fallacies

In order to successfully lose weight it's important not to fall for the following common diet misconceptions.

The Fallacy: Calories Don't Count

This is the first of the many fallacies that people use in the weight-loss business in order to convince you to try their gimmicks. On the contrary, calories do count in a weight-loss program. In order to lose a pound of fat, you must reduce your intake by 3,500 calories. However, in a low-fat, moderate lean protein and moderate complex carbohydrate diet there is no need to count calories, since by nature this is a low-calorie diet.

The Fallacy: Crash Diet to Jump-Start Weight Loss

This is probably the worst way to begin a diet program because most crash diets, which are usually low in carbohydrates, produce rapid fluid loss. This fluid loss has nothing to do with the amount of liquid a person drinks, and only reflects a change in the body's ability to hold fluid. Fat is not coming off in this type of program and, in fact, protein can be lost during a crash diet, which may be harmful to the kidneys. When these diets are abandoned, weight is gained rapidly, usually in the form of fat, and the dieter may wind up with more fat than when he or she started.

The Fallacy: Exercise Is Not Essential to Weight Loss

Nothing can be further from the truth. Regular physical exercise and activity is a key point in a long-term weight-reduction and weight-maintenance program. Exercise not only burns calories, but also has an appetite-regulating effect on the brain. Exercise also favorably affects the metabolism by lowering blood pressure, blood cholesterol, blood sugar, and, in general, contributing to good health.

The Fallacy: Anything That You Eat in the Evening Will Turn to Fat

It doesn't make any difference when you eat. It's the total number of calories you consume daily versus the total number of calories you burn daily that determines weight loss or weight gain. Your body does not differentiate calories eaten during the day or in the evening, only how many calories you have eaten on that particular day. The only disadvantage to eating late in the evening is if you have a condition known as acid reflux, and in that particular case, this could precipitate heartburn. If you do have reflux, it is certainly essential to have this checked by your physician.

The Fallacy: Certain Foods Can Burn Up Calories

As explained in Tips 6 and 10, the digestion of some foods does consume more energy than that of others, but there is no food that expends enough energy during digestion to promote any substantial weight loss by itself, without other changes to your eating and exercise habits.

The Fallacy: It Doesn't Make a Difference How Fast You Eat

Eating a meal slowly and chewing the food thoroughly gives the appetite-regulating center in the brain a chance to register what you have eaten and reduce the appetite and make you more satisfied with less food. Eating rapidly does not by itself cause you to be overweight; however, since people who eat rapidly do not give the appetite suppressing mechanism time to work, they tend to eat more.

The Fallacy: Because Meat Is High in Protein, It Doesn't Cause Weight Gain

Protein, no matter what the source, contains 4 calories per gram. Carbohydrates also contain 4 calories per gram. Fat, however, contains 9 calories per gram, more than twice as many calories as a gram of protein or carbohydrate. Meat not only gives 4 calories per gram for its protein content, but it also gives 9 calories per gram for its fat content. The greater the percentage of fat in the meat, the higher the caloric value.

Because consumption of any excessive calories above the body's metabolic requirements results in increased storage of fat, eating meat not only can cause weight gain, but can cause a greater proportion of fat to be deposited in the body because of its high fat content.

The Fallacy: As Long as You Take Your Vitamins, It Doesn't Matter What You Eat

Vitamin supplements will not provide all the daily requirements of protein, carbohydrates, minerals, amino acids, and essential fatty acids that the body needs. This is a widespread misconception about

nutrition and dieting. Many complications have been noted in people on very low-calorie diets combined with protein-vitamin supplements because of the inability of the body's metabolism,
particularly the kidneys and liver, to adjust to this type of diet.

The Fallacy: If You Skip Breakfast and Lunch and Eat a Large Dinner, You'll Lose Weight

No matter when the calories are consumed in a given twenty-four-
hour period, the end result is the same. The basic formula is calories
consumed versus calories expended. Whether you eat 400 calories
three times a day or 1,200 calories at one meal, the body does not
know the difference as far as weight gain goes. In addition, skipping
meals is not a healthful way to embark on a diet program because
the appetite becomes overstimulated late in the day and you not only
eat a large dinner, but you also eat continuous snacks through the
evening.

Tip 66 Don't Yo-Yo Diet

Yo-yo dieting or weight cycling makes it harder to permanently lose weight and is much more dangerous to your health. The Framingham Heart Study, which has followed more than five thousand people for almost forty years, recently indicated a health hazard for chronic dieters. People who lost 10 percent of their body weight had an almost 20 percent reduction in the incidence of heart disease. But when these same dieters gained back the 10 percent of their body weight, they raised their heart disease risk by almost 30 percent. So if you weighed 160 pounds and lost 10 percent, or 16 pounds, you would decrease your heart disease risk by 20 percent. But if you gained back those 16 pounds, you would increase your risk of heart attack by 30 percent, an overall net gain of 10 percent, and you would still weigh the same 160 pounds.

Experts in the fields of physiology, biochemistry, psychology, nutrition, and medicine have come up with the some startling findings about yo-yo dieting:

- The weight-loss/weight-gain cycle actually increases your desire for fatty foods. Animal research studies at Yale University showed that rats that had lost weight rapidly on low-calorie diets always chose more fat in their diets when given a choice between fat, protein, and carbohydrates. These rats always put on more weight than when they started, and in a much shorter time than it had taken them to lose the weight.
- Yo-yo dieters increase the ratio of body fat to lean body tissue with repeated bouts of weight gain and weight loss. Women who lose weight rapidly on a low-carbohydrate, high-protein diet can lose a significant amount of muscle tissue. If the weight is regained again, they usually regain more

fat and less muscle because it is easier for the body to gain fat than it is to rebuild muscle tissue.

- After yo-yo dieting, body fat gets redistributed into the abdomen from the thighs, buttocks, and hips. Medical research has shown that fat deposits above the waist increase the risk of heart disease and diabetes, not to mention that they form an unsightly paunch.

- When you lose weight by cutting calories, your basal metabolic rate (BMR) slows down because it is the body's defense mechanism against starvation. The body can't tell the difference between starvation and low-calorie dieting; consequently, your body is trying to conserve energy by burning fewer calories. This is why it becomes harder to lose weight after a week or two even though you are eating exactly the same amount of calories as you did when you first started your diet. This slowdown in the basal metabolic rate persists even after the diet is over and accounts for the rapid-rebound, excessive weight gain that dieters experience when they go off a diet. This slowdown in metabolic rate can occur even after a single attempt at dieting. However, the repeated effects of yo-yo dieting can affect the basal metabolic rate much more, making additional weight loss almost impossible and rebound weight gain almost inevitable. The yo-yo dieter is often heard to say, "I'm heavier now than I was before I started this stupid diet."

- An enzyme called *lipoprotein lipase* (LPL) becomes more active when you cut calories. This enzyme controls the amount of fat that is stored in your body's fat cells. Dieting therefore makes the body more efficient at storing fat, which is exactly the opposite of what a dieter wants. As you reduce your calorie intake, the LPL starts to activate the fat-storing process. This is another defense mechanism that the body uses to prevent starvation. Remember, the enzyme LPL doesn't know that you are dieting; it thinks you are starving to death.

• Female dieters who exhibited repeated cycles of weight gain and weight loss showed an increased risk of sudden death from heart attacks, according to a recent medical report. This study followed fifteen hundred women who had engaged in cyclic dieting over a period of twenty-five years.

■ Yo-Yo Diets and the Immune System

In addition to being bad for your waistline, yo-yo diets may also actually harm the immune system. In a study reported in the June 2004 issue of the *Journal of the American Dietetic Association*, women who had a history of repeatedly losing and regaining weight had weaker immune systems than women who did not engage in yo-yo dieting. Those women who reported losing and regaining weight more than five times over a period of years were found to have one-third fewer natural killer cells, which are essential for the body's immune system to kill viruses and bacteria.

So instead of trying every fad diet that comes along and falling into the dangerous yo-yo diet cycle, opt for a more sensible approach to dieting that combines healthy eating habits with a regular exercise program.

Tip 67 Don't Be Tempted by These Diet-Wrecking Foods

Here's a list of some of the most common diet-sabotaging foods. Next time you're tempted by one of these, opt for a healthier, lower-fat alternative:

Red Meat

Red meat, which is high in cholesterol and saturated fats, is really bad for your arteries. The fat content blocks up the coronary arteries leading to the heart, causing heart disease. It also causes the arteries in the brain to clog up, leading to strokes or TIAs (mini-strokes). The high fat content in meat has also been implicated in the development of cancer of the colon, breast, and prostate gland.

With the added hormones and potential contaminants (such as mad cow disease), red meat is about the worst food you can consume. You can get the same protein value without the added fat or detrimental compounds by substituting fish, chicken or turkey breast, beans, nuts, and soy-based foods for the fat-laden red meat.

Potato Chips and French Fries

Potato chips are high in saturated fat, trans fats, and salt. These crunchy morsels can provide the body with dangerous levels of omega-6 fatty acids, which can cause your arteries to clog up and can also cause inflammation in the body's tissues and organs. And fat may not be the only danger lurking in the ever-popular french fries. Besides saturated fats, trans fats, and tons of calories, a new hidden danger has been discovered in french fries. A recent study has found that frying or baking starchy carbohydrates like potatoes at high temperatures produces a chemical known as *acrylamide*, which is known to cause cancer and reproductive problems in laboratory animals. Many researchers feel that acrylamide poses a real cancer threat in humans.

Fast Foods

Fast foods are really bad foods, especially those sold in fast-food restaurants. One meal consisting of a double cheeseburger, large fries, and large soda is filled with enough calories, fat, sugar, and salt to raise your blood cholesterol and blood pressure and blood sugar to astronomical numbers. For healthier on-the-go alternatives, check out Tip 81.

Avoid Eating Fast-Food Fast

If you're a fast-eating fast-food eater, you're doing even more damage to your body than when you eat fast food slowly. When you consume food at a rapid pace, you have a greater tendency to consume excess calories by overeating. The reason for this is that it takes fifteen to twenty minutes for the brain's appetite regulator to receive the signals that your stomach is full. If you eat your meal rapidly in five or ten minutes, as people often do in fast-food restaurants, your appestat will not yet know that you've eaten.

You'll still be as hungry as you were before you wolfed down that bacon double cheeseburger, and you may order a milk shake and a large order of french fries. By the time you get those down the hatch, your brain will just be receiving the first signals that you're full from the double bacon cheeseburger you ate in the first five minutes. Well, it's too late by then. The appestat will never know that you've eaten 620 calories and 38 grams of fat (bacon double cheeseburger), and 590 calories and 30 grams of fat (large french fries), and 400 calories and 9 grams of fat (milk shake). Only your waistline, hips, and thighs will be the wiser.

Desserts

Most desserts, including cakes, pies, candies, and ice cream, are extremely high in refined sugar. This refined sugar content quickly increases your blood glucose level, which just as quickly increases your pancreas's production of insulin, which in turn stores excess fat in your body's cells. What happens subsequently is a rapid drop in blood sugar and an increase in your hunger level, which causes you to binge on highly refined sugar products.

Avoid rich bakery foods such as muffins, doughnuts, sweet rolls, and cakes. Most of these bakery foods contain over 50 percent fat calories in addition to the extremely high content of refined sugar. Snacks such as gingersnap cookies, angel food cake, and fruits of all shapes, sizes, and colors will satisfy your sweet tooth without adding excess sugar or fat to your diet. For more healthy dessert alternatives, see Tips 31, 46, and 82.

Be careful of the so-called diet cakes, pies, muffins, and cookies that state they are low-fat. These products usually have extremely high sugar content and an abundance of calories, and they may also contain partially hydrogenated vegetable oils and trans fats. These highly refined sweets have essentially no fiber, no nutrients, and no beneficial contents other than empty calories and should be eliminated from any real diet plan.

Smoked and Cured Fish and Meats and Pickled Foods

Smoked foods contain many harmful chemicals such as phenols and nitrates. When cooked and digested, these chemicals form nitrosamines, which are cancer-causing agents. These foods are also high in saturated fats, which can increase your risk for heart disease. Pickled foods also contain nitrates, which are converted to cancer-forming nitrosamines in the digestive tract.

Fruits and vegetables that are rich in vitamins C and A, beta-carotene, and antioxidants may be able to inhibit the formation of these cancer-causing nitrosamines. So if you have occasion to eat smoked or cured meats and fish or pickled foods, be sure to add generous amounts of veggies and fruits to your meal to counteract the harmful effects of these bad chemicals.

Salt

The National Academy of Sciences now recommends that you limit your salt or sodium intake to no more than 2,000 mg per day. Although some salt is essential in the diet for maintaining the fluid balance of the body, excess salt intake can cause a permanent elevation of blood pressure by interfering with the kidneys' ability to eliminate salt from the body. This excess accumulation of sodium causes the body to retain more liquid and subsequently increases the volume of blood. This makes the heart work harder, causing a rise in blood pressure. In susceptible people, this may result in permanent hypertension and premature death from strokes or heart attacks.

Alcohol

Excess alcohol can cause liver disease, brain damage, nerve disorders, strokes, heart disease, hypertension, damage to the reproductive organs, enlargement of the spleen, hemorrhages of the esophagus, and liver and pancreatic cancer. While a small glass of red wine daily has been shown to be heart-protective, excess alcohol can lead to many diseases and premature death. And don't forget, alcohol contains 7 calories per gram. So excessive alcohol intake is detrimental to both your health and your waistline.

Caffeine

Excess caffeine consumption causes marked fatigue after the initial stimulating effect of the caffeine wears off. Caffeine also has an adverse effect on the cardiovascular and nervous systems. It can cause a rapid heartbeat, palpitations, elevation of blood pressure, and an irritation of all of the body's nerve endings. This can result in headaches, nervousness, sweats, tremors, mental confusion, anxiety, and even paranoid behavior. Following these adverse effects is marked lethargy, which saps the body of its vital energy. One or two cups of coffee or tea daily, however, probably will not cause any of these nasty side effects, provided you do not have an exaggerated reaction to caffeine. Remember also that excess caffeine intake has an appetite-stimulating effect.

Tip 68 Don't Be Tempted by Quick-Fix Fad Diets

The diet shelf is full of fad diets that promise incredible weight loss in minimal time. They all sound too good to be true. Well, they probably are! Take the low-carb plans that stress low-carb, high-fat, high-protein diets. These diets promise weight loss from a calorie intake that is up to 60 percent fat. In addition, these diets put no restriction on the type of fat, whether it's saturated, unsaturated, or from foods that are high in cholesterol. At the same time, they restrict nutritious fruits, vegetables, cereals, beans, and whole grains that are essential for good health.

While these low-carbohydrate diets can promote short-term weight loss, rebound weight gain occurs after the initial weight loss from the unhealthy breakdown of fat and protein for fuel and depleted stores of carbohydrates. Once your body becomes aware that it is carbohydrate-depleted and exhibits the symptoms of fatigue, malaise, and muscle cramps, your brain's control center receives stress signals from all of your body's cells suffering from carbohydrate depletion. Your brain's hunger center then has no other option but to set you off on a carbohydrate binge to replace the carbohydrates needed by all of the body's cells.

What follows is rebound weight gain until your need for refined carbohydrates gets satisfied and you begin to resume your former unhealthy diet of excess fat and low carbohydrates. Rebound weight gain occurs in over 90 percent of the people who go off of these boring, dangerous, low-carb, high-fat, high-protein diets. In most cases, these individuals gain back almost all of their original weight, and some dieters even gain back more weight than they had originally lost. Not a pretty picture, is it?

Your diet should not be restricted to any one food source if you want to lose weight safely. A healthy diet should consist of approximately 60 percent complex carbohydrates, 25 percent protein, and 15 percent fat. Remember that each gram of protein and carbohydrates contains 4 calories, whereas each gram of fat contains 9 calories. You do the math! The next fad diet might seem like a great idea when you shed pounds at an unheard-of rate, but all such diets are bound to hurt your diet and health efforts in the long run.

Tip 69 Don't Join the Low-Carb Craze

The low-carbohydrate diet craze, which is essentially a high-fat, high-protein, low-carbohydrate diet, is a component of practically every diet book that has been on the market for the past ten years. These diets say that you can have bacon and eggs for breakfast, hot dogs for lunch, and a juicy steak for dinner. Sounds tempting, doesn't it? They also tell you that you can't have any, or at the very least, minimal amounts of carbohydrates with each meal; for instance, no vegetables, fruits, cereals, breads, potatoes, pasta, or grains. Sound unappetizing and unhealthy? It certainly is.

The simple fact is that you do lose weight initially on these very low-carbohydrate, high-fat, high-protein diets; however, most of the initial weight loss is water weight loss due to a metabolic process called *ketosis*, a condition usually found only in people with diseases such as diabetes and kidney disorders, not in healthy people. Once the body gets rid of this water, it starts burning fat. This, in itself, is a good thing; however, the downside is that this abnormal process of ketosis also begins to burn the body's protein, or muscle. By attempting to burn protein as a source of fuel for energy, the body is actually breaking down one of the most important elements in the body, one that is necessary for building and repairing the body's tissues, cells, and organs and sustaining life. This is one of the reasons that fatigue and general weakness have been reported as early side effects of this completely unhealthy diet.

This diet also strips the body of essential sodium and potassium, vital minerals that are essential for good health. At the same time, blood cholesterol rises dangerously, levels of thyroid hormone decrease, and the metabolism slows down to conserve energy, which slows the process of weight loss. Kidney and liver damage may result if too much of the body's protein is broken down in these diets. Without glucose to fuel the brain and nervous system, which use approximately two-thirds of the glucose present in the body, the brain's blood supply of glucose is limited, resulting in compromised brain functioning.

As you can see, this is a dangerous diet and is not healthy to remain on for any extended period of time. In addition, once this diet is stopped, rapid weight gain resumes because the body has been depleted of carbohydrates, water, and nutrients. The hunger center in the brain increases your appetite, and you usually begin to consume massive quantities of carbohydrates to alleviate the adverse effects of this diet.

Tip 70   Don't Count Carbs; Count Fat Grams

A study presented at the North American Association for the Study of Obesity in 2004 showed that low-fat diets work better at keeping weight off than low-carbohydrate diets. This study used the National Weight Control Registry that evaluated more than twenty-five hundred people between the ages of forty and fifty from 1995 to 2003 to learn how people who lost thirty or more pounds and kept them off for at least one year did it. Physicians compared diets to see if one type made a difference in amount of weight lost and then regained one year later.

The type of diet (low-fat or low-carb) made no difference in how much weight people lost initially. In fact, many of the dieters had lost an average of fifty to sixty pounds initially. However, those individuals on the low-carbohydrate diet who increased their fat intake over the next year regained the most weight. These low-carb dieters ate fewer carbohydrates while keeping the amount of protein in their diets the same. Instead of replacing carbohydrates with more protein, these low-carb dieters replaced the carbohydrates with additional fat in their diets. This increase in dietary fat resulted in the low-carb dieters regaining almost all of the weight that they had originally lost. The low-fat dieters, on the other hand, only regained 35 percent of the weight they had lost.

Other studies have also shown that low-carb dieters eventually regain all or most of the weight they have originally lost. More than one-half of Americans who have tried low-carb diets have given up, according to a recent survey. The American Institute for Cancer Research used these trends to issue a statement in September 2004 urging dieters to "come back to common sense" and eat a balanced diet by increasing fruits, vegetables, and whole grains, reducing portion size, and increasing physical activity.

Tip 71 Don't Fall for the Net Carb Scam

Net carbs, or nonimpact carbs, are popular with low-carb diets and dieters. The net carbs of a food product are the number of grams of carbs contained in that particular food minus the carbs from artificial sweeteners and fiber. The concept is that the carbs from fiber, artificial sweeteners, and sugar alcohols don't count as carbs because they do not cause spikes in blood sugar that cause an increase in your appetite.

For instance, a popular brand of cake lists the net carbs as 8 grams on the ingredients label; however, when you turn the box over and read the nutritional facts, you will see that the product actually contains 20 grams of carbs. Where did the other 12 grams of carbs disappear to? The label states that 4 grams are fiber and 8 grams are sugar alcohol. The fiber, they say, is deducted because it mostly goes through the intestinal tract without being absorbed. That's true, however, only for insoluble fiber, not soluble fiber, which is absorbed.

Sugar alcohol is also excluded from net carbs based on the idea that it has minimal impact on your blood sugar and therefore shouldn't be considered a true carbohydrate. Sugar alcohol is neither sugar nor alcohol. It's a bulking and sweetening agent used to add texture and taste to food. It still is a carbohydrate, however, and as such turns to glucose in your bloodstream. This glucose in turn stimulates the pancreas to produce additional amounts of insulin. It only takes a small increase in the level of blood insulin to keep the fat cells from releasing their fat.

As you can see, it is the total amount of carbohydrates contained in the food, not the "net carbs," that determines the body's ability to burn fat or store carbs as fat. The bottom line is really the total number of calories you consume daily, which is an accurate predictor of weight loss or weight gain. Counting carbs, whether they are real carbs or net carbs, has nothing whatsoever to do with losing real weight or maintaining weight loss. There have been no studies that prove that low net carb foods help people lose weight. Also, the Food and Drug Administration doesn't regulate using the term "net carbs" on labels, nor does it check the different carbs that food producers subtract to arrive at their magical net carb value.

So forget about counting carbs or worrying about "net carbs" when you shop for foods. Concentrate on healthy foods that are low in calories and low in fat. Choose foods that contain lean protein, with moderate amounts of fiber in the form of complex carbohydrates. Concentrate on net calories lost from your diet, not bogus net carbs on food labels.

Tip 72 Don't Try Diet Aids or Supplements

Dietary supplements, herbs, powders, pills, and drinks that contain ephedrine-type compounds known as *ephedra*, or the Chinese herb ma huang, are dangerous to your health. Ephedra is contained in a variety of diet pills and supplements that make false claims that they can aid weight loss, increase energy, and improve athletic performance. The many side effects that are related to ephedra and ephedra-like compounds include high blood pressure, increased heart rate, strokes, seizures, cardiac arrhythmias, psychotic episodes, dizziness, insomnia, psychosis, dementia, uterine contractions, and even death.

Some states have already banned the sale of these compounds in all consumer products. The American Medical Association has recently recommended that the Food and Drug Administration ban these drugs nationwide because of the serious risk factors associated with them, and the FDA has announced plans to ban the sale of all dietary supplements containing ephedra.

Compounds That Contain Ephedra

The following common compounds contain ephedra:

- Ephedrine
- Ma huang or cao ma huang (Chinese ephedra)
- Mahuuanggen
- Muzei mu huang (Mongolian ephedra)
- Natural Ecstasy
- Pinellia
- Popotillo

- Sea grape
- Sida cordifolia
- Yellow astringent
- Yellow horse
- Zhong ma huang
- Epitonin
- Herbal phen–fen
- ECA Stack

The following teas are made with the American species of ephedra:

- Brigham tea
- Mexican tea
- Squaw tea
- Desert tea
- Mormon tea
- Teamster's tea

All Diet Pills Are Bogus

Dietary aids that claim they are "fat burners," "carbohydrate busters," "starch blockers," and "muscle builders" are all bogus. They are completely without merit, and in some cases they contain a substance called *creatinine*, which can cause kidney damage. Some of these aids can have a laxative effect, and instead of losing weight, you will lose essential vitamins, nutrients, minerals, and electrolytes from your body. Some of these bogus diet aids also contain caffeine, which acts as a stimulant and can cause nervousness, palpitations, sweating, diarrhea, anxiety, and insomnia and does not help to cause weight loss. Many of these products contain a combination of herbs, starch fillers, and food dyes that are mixed with a variety of vitamins and minerals that do nothing but give you indigestion and heartburn.

If a supplement states that you can lose a lot of weight in a short period of time, you can rest assured that it is without merit. There is big money being made in the diet business, especially in diet supplements and so-called weight-loss pills. Diet promoters who make these unrealistic promises are nothing but fast-talking marketing charlatans, who hope that you will buy their products before you realize that they are bogus.

Prescription Diet Pills

The FDA is currently considering taking a popular prescription diet medication off the market because it has amphetamine-like qualities. Amphetamine drugs are extremely dangerous to your health because they can cause high blood pressure, abnormal heart rhythms, heart attacks, and strokes.

Let's put it this way: there are no safe diet pills, whether they're over-the-counter pills or those prescribed by a physician. The only way to safely lose weight is to eat less, especially less fat, and to exercise more.

PART 8

Try These Meals and Fat-Melting Tips in the Kitchen and On the Go

Tip 73 Eat These Healthy Breakfasts

It's important to make healthful choices when you start the day. Try these nutritious breakfasts:

- 1 slice cinnamon French toast made with egg substitute and whole wheat bread
- 1 cup fat-free yogurt with fresh fruit and 1 tablespoon wheat germ
- 1 nonfat waffle with fresh fruit topping
- 1 toasted small whole wheat bagel with 1 teaspoon nonfat cream cheese
- 1 cup cooked oatmeal with cinnamon and ¼ cup raisins
- 1 cup cold bran or whole wheat cereal with ½ cup fresh fruit
- 1 poached, fried, or scrambled egg (cooked with nonfat spray) with 1 slice whole wheat toast or oat bran or whole wheat English muffin with 1 teaspoon all-fruit jam
- Omelet made with 2 egg whites or egg substitute with 1 slice low-fat or skim milk cheese, tomato, onion, green pepper, and/or mushrooms
- 1 scooped-out whole wheat bagel with 1 slice unsalted smoked salmon (nova lox) with nonfat cream cheese, tomato, and onion
- 2 small whole wheat or buckwheat pancakes made with egg substitute, topped with fresh fruit and/or sugar-free syrup
- 1 fried egg (cooked with nonfat spray) and 2 small nonfat veggie sausages or 2 slices nonfat turkey bacon

Tip 74 Love These
Slimming Lunches

A filling, nutritious lunch is important. Here are some great healthy, diet-friendly options:

- Veggie burger on whole wheat bread or bun with lettuce, tomato, onion, and ketchup
- Peanut butter and jelly sandwich made with 1 tablespoon reduced-fat peanut butter and 1 tablespoon jelly on whole wheat bread
- Veggie cream cheese sandwich made with 2 tablespoons non-fat cream cheese on whole wheat bread with sprouts, tomato, cucumber, and lettuce
- Cream cheese and jelly sandwich made with 2 tablespoons nonfat cream cheese and 1 tablespoon jelly on whole wheat bread
- Tuna pita sandwich made with 1 medium whole wheat pita pocket and 3 ounces tuna (packed in water) with lettuce, tomato, cucumber, sprouts, and 1 teaspoon Dijon mustard or nonfat mayonnaise.
- Chicken pita sandwich made with 1 medium whole wheat pita pocket with 3 ounces grilled chicken breast and 1 teaspoon nonfat mayonnaise with lettuce, tomato, celery, and cucumber
- Cheese sandwich made with 2 slices skim milk cheese (such as Alpine Lace) or other low-fat cheese with 1 teaspoon mustard or nonfat mayonnaise and lettuce, tomato, shredded carrots, and sprouts on whole wheat bread

- Turkey sandwich made with 2 slices reduced-fat turkey breast with 1 teaspoon mustard or nonfat mayonnaise, lettuce, and tomato on a whole wheat bun
- 1 cup minestrone, lentil, split pea, or any vegetable or bean-based soup with 1 small whole wheat roll
- 1 soft corn tortilla with ⅓ cup fat-free refried beans and shredded low-fat cheese, lettuce, tomato, and salsa
- 12 steamed mussels or clams with ½ cup marinara sauce and 1 small whole wheat roll
- Chicken Caesar salad made with lettuce, tomato, chopped celery, cucumber, 3 ounces grilled chicken breast, nonfat Parmesan cheese, and 2 tablespoons fat-free Caesar dressing
- Veggie hoagie made with ½ scooped-out Italian roll and your choice of tomatoes, lettuce, olives, peppers, onions, cucumbers, carrots, and/or sprouts
- 1 whole wheat bagel (scooped out) with 1 slice smoked salmon (nova lox) and tomato, onion, and lettuce
- Grilled cheese sandwich made with 1 whole wheat bagel (scooped out), 2 slices low-fat cheese, 1 teaspoon Dijon mustard or nonfat mayonnaise, and tomato
- 3 ounces sardines (drained) on whole wheat bread or pita with tomato, lettuce, and onion
- 1 slice light cheese pizza topped with veggies of your choice and a side salad with 2 tablespoons nonfat dressing
- Nicoise salad with mixed greens, tuna, string beans, tomato, anchovies, ½ sliced hard-boiled egg, olives, radishes, celery, onions, and bell pepper with mustard vinaigrette dressing on the side (dip fork in dressing sparingly) and one scooped-out French roll

Tip 75 Try These Healthy, No-Hassle Dinners

Coming up with creative dinner ideas can be a struggle, let alone trying to come up with waist-friendly dinners. Here's a list of easy-to-make, appetite-pleasing dinners to try:

- 1 grilled 3-ounce, lean hamburger on a small whole wheat roll with lettuce, tomato, onion, and ketchup and 1 small white potato made into oven-baked french fries (slice into fries, spray nonstick pan with nonfat spray, and bake at 400° until crisp).
- ½ cup fat-free baked beans, 1 nonfat beef hot dog or turkey dog on a small whole wheat bun with sauerkraut, relish, and mustard, and small side salad with 2 tablespoons nonfat dressing
- 3 ounces sardines (drained) or tuna (packed in water) in large tossed salad of lettuce or Romaine, tomato, cucumber, pepper, onion, sprouts, carrots, and olives with 2 tablespoons nonfat dressing or mustard vinaigrette dressing
- 1 cup spinach fettuccine with fresh vegetables with ½ cup tomato or marinara sauce and large tossed salad
- 1 cup whole wheat spaghetti with 12 clams or mussels, garlic, ⅓ cup white wine, 1 teaspoon olive oil, and seasoning and large tossed salad
- 3-ounce grilled salmon steak or salmon fillet with tomatoes, onions, peppers, and garlic, small baked potato or yam with skin, and 1 cup steamed vegetable of your choice
- 1 cup Chinese greens with 6 medium grilled shrimp and garlic with 1 cup brown rice

- 2 soft tacos with nonfat refried beans, 3 ounces sliced grilled chicken, lettuce, tomato, onion, grated nonfat cheese, and salsa
- 3 ounces lean roast beef with horseradish, small baked potato or yam with skin, 1 cup steamed veggies, and 1 small whole wheat roll
- 6 medium shrimp with cocktail sauce, 1 small ear of corn, and 1 cup steamed asparagus, broccoli, or spinach
- 3 ounces broiled or baked cod, halibut, mackerel, or sole with grilled onions, peppers, mushrooms, and tomatoes, cooked with lemon, wine, and seasonings, 1 small whole wheat roll, and tossed salad
- 2 small lamb chops (trim fat) with 2 teaspoons mint jelly and whole broiled tomato, 1 small baked sweet potato, and tossed salad
- Goat cheese salad made with reduced-fat goat cheese, mixed greens, tomato, olives, bell peppers, cucumber, and celery with mustard vinaigrette dressing on the side (dip fork in dressing sparingly) and 1 scooped-out Italian or French roll
- Spinach salad with 1 ounce low-fat blue cheese, ½ ounce chopped walnuts, sliced apples, cherry tomatoes, cucumbers, and 1 tablespoon dressing (made with 1 tablespoon Dijon mustard, 1 teaspoon olive oil, lemon juice from ½ lemon—squeezed—or lemon zest)
- 1 cup low-fat macaroni and cheese with 1 cup zucchini, diced tomatoes, onions, and garlic, 1 ear of corn or a small sweet potato, and ½ cup steamed fresh carrots

Tip 76 Season with Garlic and Onions

You don't have to cook with tons of fats and oil to flavor your foods. Garlic and onions contain phytonutrients that break down fat globules from food in the intestinal tract, preventing this fat from being absorbed into the body. Less fat absorbed means less fat stored in your fat cells, which translates into less weight gained. Garlic and onions also help reduce your appetite.

In addition to these fat-busting properties, the phytonutrients in garlic help reduce the incidence of heart disease and have been shown to inactivate certain viruses that cause intestinal and respiratory illnesses. Onions contain a phytonutrient called quercetin that has been shown to keep blood from clotting by reducing the stickiness of the blood platelets. This helps reduce the risk of heart attacks and strokes.

And besides the health benefits, both garlic and onion make for fabulous seasonings to your favorite dishes—enjoy!

Tip 77 Try a Salad Sandwich

For a lower-calorie lunch alternative, try an egg, tuna, or chicken salad sandwich with a twist: a bread-free sandwich. Take a large piece of iceberg or Romaine lettuce and use it as a wrap with your favorite salad ingredients. It's more fun than a traditional salad, and you get the crunch factor of eating a sandwich without the added calories of bread! Salad sandwiches are low in calories and high in nutrition. Here's one instance when even a second helping won't interfere with your weight-loss program.

The salad sandwich possibilities are endless. Using lettuce in place of bread will convert your favorite turkey, chicken, or cheese sandwich into a diet powerhouse. Add sliced tomato or cucumber to improve the texture, taste, and crunch of your salad sandwich. Tuna, chicken, crab meat, and egg salads also make tasty, nutritious, low-calorie, high-protein lettuce wraps.

To keep your salad sandwich low in fat, make sure you prepare them using nonfat or very low-fat mayo. Try spicing your chicken salad up with a little Indian curry powder, lemongrass and lime, or add grapes, pecans, walnuts, and apples for flavor. Crab salad can also be made with lemon juice, watercress, Dijon mustard, and a touch of olive oil. When making egg salad, try using two or three fresh hard-boiled eggs and discarding the yolk from one of them. This lowers the cholesterol count without reducing the taste of the egg salad. Chop in some fresh dill and celery to boost the taste.

■ The Incredible Egg

Egg yolk is not as bad as it was once thought to be. Egg yolk contains two chemicals called lutein and xanthine that are important in shielding the retina of the eye from the harmful effects of ultraviolet light from the sun. These two chemicals also appear to reduce the risk of both developing cataracts and macular degeneration of the eye. Since eggs are low in saturated fat, there appears to be no direct link between the cholesterol content of egg yolk and heart disease. Eggs are also low in calories and are chock-full of nutrition, including protein and vitamins A and B_{12}, folic acid, and riboflavin. For good nutrition and weight loss, eat an egg every other day and on alternate days eat two egg whites from hard-boiled eggs or make an egg white omelet with fresh veggies.

Tip 78 Mix and Match for a Fat-Melting Salad

Here are some healthy, nutritious salad ingredients that are low in calories and fat, contain good sources of protein, and are packed with vitamins, minerals, and phytonutrients. You can mix and match any of these ingredients, or any other similar salad ingredients, for your really good salad.

- 1 cup Boston lettuce or baby spinach (30 calories, high in vitamin K and folate)
- 3 tablespoons (¼ cup) raisins (70 calories, 2 grams fiber, 310 mg potassium, 0 grams fat)
- 1 tablespoon roasted sunflower or sesame seeds or walnuts (40 calories, 3 grams good fat, 1 gram fiber, 100 IU vitamin E)
- ⅓ cup tofu cubes (30 calories, 1 gram fat, 10 mg iron)
- ⅓ cup sliced carrots (10 calories, 0 grams fat, high in vitamin A, B, and carotene)
- ⅓ cup broccoli (10 calories, 0 grams fat, high in vitamin K)
- 1 tablespoon feta cheese (25 calories, 2 gram fat, 50 mg calcium)
- ⅓ cup sliced beets (10 calories, 0 grams fat, 1 gram fiber)
- ⅓ cup chickpeas (48 calories, 0.5 grams fat, 1 gram fiber, good source of vitamins B_6 and B_{12})
- ⅓ cup alfalfa sprouts (3 calories, 0 grams fat, 0.5 grams fiber)
- 1 sliced egg white (20 calories, 0 grams fat, good source of protein and vitamin D)
- 2 medium black olives (21 calories, 4 grams good olive oil fat, 1 gram fiber)

Add a sliced chicken breast or a small can of tuna packed in water to the salad to make it an entire meal packed with lean protein.

Tip 79 Tips for Eating Well While Eating Out

It goes without saying that you have more control over the fat and calorie content of your meals when you make them yourself. But just because you are dining out doesn't mean you have to give up on your diet. Here are some tips to keep your fat and calorie intake in check at restaurants and social events:

• Always choose lower-fat foods such as broiled fish or chicken without fattening sauces. As a side dish, you can have a large tossed salad with the dressing on the side.

• Many restaurants cook their vegetables with added fats, so that veggie appetizer you ordered might not be as healthy as you think! Be sure to ask how vegetables will be prepared, or request steamed veggies without additional fats or sauces.

• Don't be afraid to send back your meal in a restaurant if they didn't follow your instructions for your order. For example, if you asked for steamed vegetables, baked potato, and broiled fish without butter, that's the way it should arrive on your plate.

• At parties, weddings, and other social events, concentrate on the fresh vegetables, without the dips, and fresh fruits. Avoid those fat-laden little appetizers with toothpicks in them. The toothpicks are red flags warning you to stay away!

• Avoid drinking excess alcohol at restaurants, since it can increase your appetite and add extra calories. Alcohol is also high in calories: 1 gram of alcohol contains 7 calories, higher than a gram of carbohydrate or protein. If you definitely like a drink with dinner, a wine spritzer is a good choice that is relatively low in total calories. And it is perfectly diet-friendly to have 4 ounces of red wine or a light beer three times a week.

At Your Favorite Restaurant

By following these suggestions, you can stick with your diet while still eating at your favorite restaurant:

Healthy Choices for Mexican Restaurants

When eating at Mexican restaurants, stay away from the deep-fried tortilla chips and order oven-baked chips with salsa instead. Skip the sour cream and go light on the guacamole, both of which are high in fat. Soft corn tortillas (tostados or enchiladas) with chicken, tomato sauce, and onions are good low-fat choices. Burritos or fajitas without sour cream or guacamole and with lettuce, tomato, and onion are also excellent low-fat dishes to order. Avoid regular refried beans, deep-fried chimichangas, and beef taco salad, which are all high in fat and calories.

Healthy Choices for Chinese Restaurants

While out to dinner at a Chinese restaurant, keep in mind that stir-fried foods are better than deep-fried. Choose dishes with grains and vegetables. Order brown rice instead of white rice for the extra fiber content (not fried rice, which also comes out brown in color but is low in fiber and high in fat). Opt for vegetable wonton soup or any vegetable-based soup rather than meat-based soups. Ask to have your food prepared without soy sauce or MSG.

Healthy Choices for Italian Restaurants

When dining Italian, remember that thinner noodles such as spaghetti, angel hair pasta, or linguini are low-fat alternatives to wider pastas. Stick to tomato or marinara sauces (some, however, have too much oil, and you can have the waiter drain the oil from the pasta and bring back your dish). Seafood-based sauces without cream are also good options. Avoid creamy, high-fat sauces such as alfredo. If you can, order whole-grain pasta or spinach noodles for their high fiber content.

Try ordering a cheese-free pizza (tomato pie) topped with a variety of fresh vegetables. You can sprinkle on a little Parmesan cheese for taste. If you prefer your pizza with cheese, order one with lots of vegetables to increase the fiber and nutrition. A great tip is to always blot a cheese pizza with a couple of napkins before eating to remove the extra oil and fat.

Tip 80 Sneak in More Fruits and Veggies

Most people don't get their daily servings of five fruits and vegetables. A smart trick for sneaking in your daily dose of fruits and vegetables is to add them to most any food you order or eat that doesn't come with fruits or vegetables included. Here are some good and good-for-you suggestions:

- Next time you order a waffle or pancake, get it with fruit on top. Berries, bananas, and apples are all good options. Some restaurants even give you the option of having the fruit mixed right into the batter. Next time you're deciding between the plain short stack or the blueberry pancakes, go for the fruit!
- Add green peppers, mushrooms, onions, broccoli, or spinach to your pizza.
- Add more vegetables such as peppers, mushrooms, onions, or spinach to an omelet.
- Load up any sandwich with cucumbers, tomatoes, lettuce, and sprouts.
- Add some sliced apples and pears or some grapes to your salad.
- Add some sliced banana to your peanut butter sandwich.
- Order a veggie burger instead of a meat burger.

And these are just a few suggestions to get you started. Be creative and you'll be eating five a day in no time!

Tip 81 Fast Food Doesn't Have to Be Fat Food

Most fast foods are so high in calories, saturated fats, and sodium that they not only make us fatter, but they also cause the buildup of fat in our arteries, causing heart attacks, strokes, and high blood pressure. But just because you are eating on the go doesn't mean you have to sacrifice your diet and your health. Keep this helpful list of the best and worst fast-food options handy the next time you're eating on the run.

The Best

If you have to eat on the go, here are some waist-friendlier fast food options to try:

- Choose a single hamburger without cheese or sauce. Add lettuce, tomato, and onion, with or without ketchup or nonfat mayo, skip the fries, and order a diet soda.
- Order a grilled chicken sandwich without the mayo, or better yet, a grilled chicken Caesar salad with fat-free herb vinaigrette dressing on the side.
- A good choice is a small vegetable chili without cheese.
- Try a soft chicken taco without sauce.
- Get pizza without extra cheese or meat; add fresh veggies to increase the nutrition content.
- Order a large salad plain, or with grilled chicken, and add fat-free dressing on the side.
- Choose a roast beef sandwich without the sauce.
- If you must have fries, order the smallest bag and either split with a friend or eat half and toss the rest.

The Worst

The following are fast food options to avoid at all costs:

- The average double cheeseburger, with large fries and a large soda, contains approximately 1,800 to 2,000 calories and approximately 100 grams of fat, of which almost 40 grams are saturated fat. It also contains approximately 1,500 mg of sodium. So, for most people, that amounts to the number of calories that they should consume in an entire day and three to four times the amount of fat and salt they should consume in a day.
- 2 slices of pizza with extra cheese and/or meat contain 750 to 800 calories, 35 to 40 grams of fat (15 grams of saturated fat), and 2,000 mg sodium.
- Fried fish sandwiches contain approximately 700 calories, 40 grams of fat (15 grams of saturated fat), and 1,200 mg sodium.
- Nachos with cheese and sour cream contain 1,200 to 1,300 calories, 80 grams fat (25 grams saturated fat), and 2,500 mg sodium.
- A chocolate milk shake contains almost 800 calories and 40 grams of fat, of which 25 grams are saturated.
- A large cola contains 200 calories.
- Large fries contain over 600 calories, 20 grams of fat, and 10 to 12 grams of saturated fat.
- Fried chicken or a fried chicken wrap with cheese and sauce contains 700 calories and 44 grams of fat (12 grams saturated fat), and 2,000 mg of sodium.

Tip 82 Know the Best of the Worst Junk Foods

Unfortunately, there are lots of times when you're placed in a position where you just can't eat healthy. What do you do if you are waiting at the airport for a flight and food selections look grim? Or maybe you are at a movie or sporting event with limited food choices. And then there are parties and work meetings. The situations are endless.

Just because you are dieting doesn't mean you have to go hungry. All you have to do is make the best choices from the worst foods. Here are some examples of the best of the worst foods.

Choosing Between Pretzels, Chips, and Mixed Nuts

Your flight lands in thirty minutes and you want to grab something quickly to tide you over until touchdown. Your options are limited and aren't looking too diet-friendly. What do you do?

Pretzels are low in fat and calories; however, they're also low in protein and fiber, so even though they're a good initial snack, you're bound to be hungry sooner. Chips are high in fat and calories and low in fiber and protein, so they are a lose-lose combination. Whether they're potato chips or corn chips or nachos, they usually have tons of fat and little nutrition value. Peanuts and other nuts are higher in fat and calories than pretzels; however, they have enough protein and fiber to keep your hunger at bay until you can get a really healthy meal. So go for the mixed nuts: they're the best of the worst.

Choosing Between a Hot Dog, a Hamburger, and a Slice of Pizza

You're enjoying an evening game at the ballpark when your friend decides to get dinner at the vendors. You're hungry, too, but don't want to break your diet. What do you do?

Both the hot dog and the hamburger are filled with lots of saturated fat; however, they do have high protein content. But who really knows what's in that hot dog or what additives and contaminants are contained in that juicy hamburger? Pizza is also high in fat and calories; however, it does contain protein and calcium from the cheese and fiber and antioxidants, particularly lycopene, in the tomato sauce. So as long as you keep it pepperoni-free, pizza is your best of the worst choice.

Choosing Between a Muffin, a Doughnut, and a Bagel with Cream Cheese

It's an early morning meeting at the office, and the breakfast options are slim, but not slimming. You know it's better to eat breakfast than skip a meal. What do you do?

Both the doughnut and muffin are loaded with fat and calories, with little or no fiber or protein, unless it is a bran muffin, which is still high in fat and calories. The cream cheese is high in fat, but provides calcium and protein. And the bagel is high in calories, but it does have some fiber, especially if there is a whole wheat bagel. So the bagel with cream cheese is your clear best of the worst choice. To make this best of the worst even better, scoop out the bagel and scrape off some of the cream cheese.

Choosing Between a Chocolate Candy Bar, Peanut Butter or Cheese Crackers, and Popcorn

You're scoping out the vending machine for a quick hunger fix, and the options look fattening and grim. What do you do?

The candy bar is loaded with lots of fat, about 10 to 15 grams, most of which is saturated fat. It also has somewhere between 250 and 300 calories, making it the biggest loser out of these three. The peanut butter and cheese crackers are high in refined carbs, fat, and calories, although not as high as the candy bar. Their only redeeming quality is 3 or 4 grams of protein. Not great, but a better choice than the candy bar. The popcorn, on the other hand, has fiber (approximately 2 grams per small bag) and is considerably lower in calories than the candy bar or peanut butter and cheese crackers. Popcorn still has plenty of carbs, but it satisfies your appetite longer because of the fiber and air bulk of the popcorn. So long as you don't add butter to it, popcorn is your best of the worst choice.

Choosing Between Cake and Ice Cream

Cake and ice cream are the most common desert options at parties. What do you do when you want to celebrate with something sweet but don't want to sabotage your diet?

Cake is packed with calories, fat, and refined sugars, with no redeeming nutritional qualities. If it has rich and gooey frosting, it's even worse for you. Ice cream is high in fat, particularly saturated fat, but it does contain calcium, potassium, and protein, making it your best of the worst choice. Opt for a low-fat scoop if it's available.

PART 9

■

Get Moving!

Tip 83 Work Out to Lose Weight

You know that in order to lose weight you need to take in fewer calories than you burn off. We've already talked about various ways to give yourself a weight-loss edge by eating healthy, low-fat foods. The other piece of the puzzle is to exercise regularly to burn off excess calories.

It's not necessary to join a gym or participate in aerobics classes to burn up fat. You can burn calories by just climbing the stairs, cleaning the house, riding a bike, working in the garden, or just by walking thirty minutes every day. You don't even have to work up a sweat to burn calories while exercising. Studies have proven that people who take a brisk walk for thirty minutes every day burn body fat, improve their physical fitness, and lower their blood pressure, as much as, if not even more than, people who work out at a gym three to four days per week. Even two fifteen-minute walks per day will give you the same fitness and fat-burning benefits as a thirty-minute walk every day.

And weight loss isn't the only reason you should get moving. A recent study from a major university showed that sedentary women, in addition to gaining weight in their abdomens, buttocks, and thighs, increased their deep fat that surrounds the internal organs of the body. This increases the risk of heart disease, hypertension, and diabetes. The study also showed that moderate exercise five times per week for thirty to forty minutes decreased the deep fat by more than 35 percent and resulted in considerable weight loss over a three-month period.

Exercise will help boost your energy as well. With the advent of the computer age, people are forced by design to do less and less physical labor. It would seem logical that this would result in more energy being available for other activities. However, how many times have you noticed that the less you do, the more tired you feel, whereas the more active you are, the more energy you have for other activities? Exercise improves the efficiency of the lungs, the heart, and the circulatory system in their ability to take in and deliver oxygen throughout the entire body. This oxygen is the catalyst that burns the fuel, food, we take in to produce energy. Consequently, the more oxygen we take in, the more energy we have for all of our activities.

Oxygen is the vital ingredient that is necessary for our survival. Since oxygen can't be stored, our cells need a continuous supply in order to remain healthy. Exercise increases your body's ability to extract oxygen from the air so that increased amounts of oxygen are available for every organ, tissue, and cell in the body. Exercise actually increases the total volume of blood, making more red blood cells available to carry oxygen and nutrition to the tissues and to remove carbon dioxide and waste products from the body's cells. This increased saturation of the tissues with oxygen is also aided by the opening of small blood vessels, which is another direct result of exercise.

So let's take that first step for energy, fitness, and real weight loss. Exercising every day—whether by walking, riding your bike to work, taking the stairs, or hitting the gym—will keep a fresh supply of oxygen surging through your blood vessels to all of your body's hungry cells. Don't disappoint these little fellows, because you depend on them as much as they depend on you. If you short-change them on their daily oxygen supply, they'll take it out on you in the form of illness and disease, but if you give them what they need, they will repay you with better health.

Tip 84 Stick with the Program

How many times have you heard someone, or even perhaps yourself, say, "I'm giving up. Exercise is boring." Over 65 percent of people who start an exercise program abandon it after four to six weeks. Surprising, isn't it? Not really. Initial enthusiasm is often quickly replaced by boredom. Most of the exercise equipment and athletic clothes people buy quickly find their way into the recesses of the closet.

The key to staying with your exercise program is to keep it fun. Exercise is not just a means to physical fitness, good health, weight control, and longevity. It is a stress-relieving, fun-filled activity. Here are some tips to keep your exercise program interesting, enjoyable, and, most of all, filled with fun, so that you'll actually be losing weight without even realizing it:

- **Don't expect results too soon.** Whether it's weight control or physical fitness that you're looking for, remember, "Rome wasn't built in a day, and neither were you." Give your body time to adapt to your regular walking program.
- **Make your exercise program convenient and flexible.** The more adaptable you are as to when and where you exercise, the more likely you are to do it on a regular basis.
- **Vary your exercise program.** Vary your exercise times (morning, afternoon, or evening) depending on your schedule.
- **Change your routine every week or two.** Try to mix up your activities to keep things interesting. Go for a long walk one afternoon or evening after work. Take your bike out for an hour or so on a weekend afternoon. Exercise doesn't have to be monotonous!

- **Record your weight only once every week.** See if you are losing the amount of weight you'd like to lose, or if you are just exercising to maintain your present weight.
- **Work out with a friend.** Exercise can be a social activity as well as good for your health. Having a workout buddy will keep exercise fun and will also help motivate you when you're feeling uninspired.
- **Don't be afraid to take a break for a few days or even a week.** Any exercise program can eventually become a little tiring. A few days' break from your schedule will give you a short breather so that you can return to your exercise program with renewed interest and enthusiasm. Remember, you won't gain all of your weight back or get out of shape if you take an occasional break.
- **Never exercise if you are injured or ill.** Your body needs time to heal and recuperate from whatever ails you. Remember, you can't exercise through an injury or an illness. Many so-called fitness nuts have tried this with disastrous results. For example, a strained muscle has been aggravated into a fractured bone or a simple cold has turned into pneumonia. Listen to your body.
- **Promise yourself a treat when you stick to your exercise program.** For example, a bouquet of flowers, a night at the theater, a movie, a ball game, a new dress, or a weekend away. Indulge yourself. You deserve it!

Tip 85 Curb Your Appetite with Exercise

Many people hesitate to start an exercise program along with their diet because they fear that exercise will stimulate their appetite, causing them to eat more. Contrary to popular belief, moderate exercise actually decreases your appetite. It does this by several mechanisms:

1. Exercise regulates the brain's appetite control center (appestat), which controls your hunger pangs. Too little exercise causes your appetite to increase by stimulating the appestat to make you hungry. Exercising, on the other hand, slows the appestat down, thus decreasing your hunger pangs.

2. Exercising redirects the blood supply away from your stomach to the exercising muscles. With less blood supplied to the stomach, your appetite is reduced.

3. Moderate exercise such as walking burns fat rather than carbohydrates and therefore does not drop the blood sugar precipitously. Strenuous exercises and very low calorie diets both drop the blood sugar rapidly, and it is this low blood sugar that stimulates your appetite and makes you hungry. Walking, on the other hand, is a more moderate type of exercise and consequently burns fats slowly, rather than carbohydrates quickly. This results in the blood sugar remaining constant. And when the blood sugar remains level, you do not feel hungry.

4. Exercising also helps to increase the resting basal metabolic rate (BMR), as explained in Tip 86. This basal metabolic rate refers to the calories your body burns at rest in order to produce energy. When you go on a calorie-restricted diet, your BMR slows down because your body assumes that the

reduction in calories is the result of starvation, so your body wants to burn fewer calories so you won't starve to death. This is one of the reasons you don't continue to lose weight on a calorie restriction diet. If, however, you are combining exercise such as walking with your diet, then the walking keeps the BMR elevated even though you are dieting. The result: less hunger and more calories burned when you walk every day.

Tip 86 Rev Up Your Metabolism with Exercise

There invariably comes a point after you've dieted and lost weight that you reach a plateau where you can't lose any more weight, no matter how hard you try. No matter how many calories you reduce from your diet, your weight doesn't budge. Being stuck at a plateau weight can be very disheartening and often may lead you to abandon your diet efforts.

The only way to break through this plateau is to increase your aerobic exercise and beef up your strength-training activity. Aerobic activities such as walking, jumping rope, dancing, tennis, and other sports, as well as indoor exercises like the treadmill, can all be part of your calorie-burning aerobic fitness activity. Aerobic exercise burns extra calories that you can't possibly lose by dieting alone. Exercising for twenty minutes a day can improve your cardiovascular fitness while you burn unwanted fat calories, which helps you break the diet plateau. In four to six weeks' time, you'll see those extra stubborn pounds melt away as you successfully move toward your target weight.

The added bonus of a regular exercise program is that you actually continue to burn calories after you stop exercising. You will continue to burn fat for many hours after your aerobic walking exercise program is finished. It takes time for the metabolic rate to slow down after exercise, which is why you can eat extra calories after walking without gaining weight.

And before your body has a chance to slow down its metabolic rate, you will be exercising again. Your body starts to get used to this higher basal metabolic rate, and therefore runs at a higher speed daily. The result: more calories burned per day, which means increased weight loss and a decrease in rebound weight gained.

The opposite is also true. Little or no exercise translates into a slower metabolic rate. This means you'll burn fewer calories than you take in and weight gain gradually ensues. Excess calories go straight to your fat storage cells, where they comfortably rest. The result, of course, is excess fat storage in your abdomen, buttocks, hips, and thighs.

Physical activity like an aerobic exercise program also cuts your appetite by suppressing the brain's appetite control center, as explained in Tip 85. The brain reasons that if you are exercising, then you shouldn't be eating. This results in less hunger, fewer calories consumed, and thus less weight gain. As you burn extra calories, you will also boost your energy level. Aerobic exercise leads to a boost in energy and an increase in endorphins, which result in a feeling of well-being. This extra energy will help you to want to continue with your aerobic exercise or walking program on a regular basis. You will not only be energetic, happy, and motivated, but you will get thin in the process.

Tip 87 Muscle Up
Your Metabolism

If you add strength-training exercises to your aerobic activity, you will begin to build muscle mass, which increases your body's metabolic rate still more. The additional lean muscle mass you develop during weight-training will help you burn calories at a faster rate even when you're at rest. One pound of lean muscle burns ten times as many calories as a pound of fat. Weight training, therefore, is an added boost that helps you lose weight and keep it off. The combination of a healthy diet, aerobic activity, and strength-training exercises will reshape your body as you lose those difficult unwanted pounds.

Studies reported at the 2004 Experimental Biology Meeting in Washington, D.C., showed that short, simple weight-training workouts helped men and women lose weight and keep that weight off permanently. Weight training also was shown to strengthen the body's immune system and lower blood pressure. By following a low-fat, moderate protein and complex carbohydrate diet, combined with simple weight-training exercises for fourteen weeks, the participants in this study lost fat and weight and increased the proportion of muscle to body weight. Also, these men and women showed significant improvements in blood pressure, heart rate, and aerobic fitness.

Another similar study showed that middle-aged and elderly people developed stronger muscles and a healthier immune system while walking regularly combined with weight-training exercises. Many of the middle-aged and elderly people in this study were moderately obese when they started the program. After twelve weeks, the majority of the obese participants had lost considerable weight, in addition to gaining lean muscle mass. These individuals also developed improved cardiovascular fitness, gained muscle strength, and boosted their energy levels.

Strength training is essential for weight control, muscle strengthening, skeletal health, and overall well-being. Strength-training exercises or using light handheld weights while walking make muscles stronger and strengthen the skeleton. The bones strengthen because the traction or tension from the contracting muscles causes the bones to absorb more calcium from the bloodstream and lose less calcium. This process increases the mineral content of the bones, thus strengthening the bones and making them less brittle as you age.

Studies show that strength-training exercises should be done two or three times per week, not on consecutive days, to prevent damage to your muscle fibers, which need time to regenerate after being stressed with weight-resistance exercises. Also, varying the muscle groups during strength-training exercises helps to provide strength benefits to all of the upper body's muscles. Newer research in exercise physiology has shown that working out a particular muscle group only twice a week offers the same strength and muscle toning benefits as working these muscles three times per week.

Many studies have shown that people who engage in strength-training exercises increase their skeletal muscle mass by approximately 1.5 kilograms (3.3 pounds), whereas sedentary people lose 0.5 kilogram (1.1 pounds) of muscle mass over a one-year period. Likewise, bone mineral density increased by 1 percent in the strength-training group and decreased by 2.5 percent in the sedentary group. Also, these studies showed that strength training in men and women increased their lean muscle mass by 4 percent and decreased their fat mass by 8 percent.

What do all these numbers mean? They mean that your muscles will become more defined and shapely and you will feel stronger because your muscles are stronger. You will have better balance and greater joint flexibility. You will feel more energetic and more confident. Your bones will be structurally stronger and less likely to break as you get older.

■ Won't Weight Training Make My Muscles Bulky?

Many women are afraid to engage in strength-training activities for fear of developing massive muscles. In reality, women don't have to be afraid they will turn into Arnold Schwarzenegger. Men start out with more muscle mass to begin with and they also bulk up more than women because they have much higher levels of testosterone in their bodies than women do. However, due to genetics and estrogen levels, most women have more body fat than men, therefore women are less likely to bulk up when weight training. Strength-training exercises increase the basal metabolic rate in women, which burns additional calories and further prevents muscles from overdeveloping. Women's muscles become more defined and sculptured, rather than bulky when they lift weights. Through strength-training exercises such as light-weight reps at the gym or walking with handheld weights, women can look forward to an overall improvement in muscle tone and strength; their muscles will become sexier, defined, and sculptured for a trim, firm look.

What's Good for Your Figure Is Good for Your Heart

Weight resistance exercises are not only good for your muscles, but are also good for the body's most important muscle—the heart. A report released by the American Heart Association in the *Journal of Circulation* in February 2000 said that there is now increasing evidence that strength training can favorably modify many risk factors for heart disease, including blood cholesterol and triglycerides, blood pressure, body fat levels, and glucose metabolism. Previously, the conventional thinking was that strength–training exercises helped to build and sculpt your muscles but did little to help the cardiovascular system and, in fact, might even be harmful to your heart. This study dispelled many of the myths and misconceptions regarding strength training. It showed that strength training is not in the least harmful if one is reasonable and not trying to be a power weight lifter.

Another related study was released in the *Journal of Hypertension*, also in February 2000. This study showed that strength-training exercises could significantly lower blood pressure. Those women who regularly lifted light weights experienced a reduction in resting systolic blood pressure (when the heart muscles contract) and a reduction in the resting diastolic blood pressure (when the heart muscles relax). Their resting blood pressures dropped regardless of their body composition, whether they performed heavy weight-resistance exercises with longer rest periods or lighter weight exercises with shorter rest periods.

Tip 88 Gain Without Pain

Exercise doesn't have to be stressful, painful, or exhausting to be beneficial; moderate exercise prevents heart disease and is a healthy component of any weight-loss or fitness plan.

In a recent study of over seventeen thousand women and men, it was concluded that moderate exercise is an independent factor in the prevention of deaths by cardiovascular diseases. The American Heart Association presented the following findings:

- Despite blood pressure, cholesterol, or age, moderate exercise has an independent effect in preventing heart disease and strokes.
- Men in the lower 20 percent of physical fitness had a 50 percent higher incidence for heart disease than men falling in the 30 to 50 percent range of fitness development.
- Women in the bottom 20 percent zone of fitness, however, had a 70 percent higher incidence of heart disease than those women in the 30 to 50 percent range of fitness development.
- The major conclusion was that "just a little bit of exercise" is all that is needed to lower your risk of cardiovascular disease.

Researchers at the Centers for Disease Control in Atlanta revealed a startling finding after reviewing forty-three previous studies on heart disease. The one statistically significant predisposing factor in the development of heart disease, which appeared in every single study, was a *lack of exercise*. Their research revealed that people who exercised the least had almost twice the risk of developing heart disease as those who exercised regularly. This particular study brought together the findings of the forty-three previous studies, which had all measured physical activity in many different ways. Walking was as effective as any other type of exercise in preventing heart disease, without the added risk of injury and disability that occurred in the more strenuous exercises. This analysis suggests that the lack of exercise on its own may be as strong a risk factor for developing heart disease as high blood pressure, smoking, and high cholesterol.

So don't concern yourself with meeting the so-called "target heart rate" during your workouts or worry whether or not you are exercising strenuously enough. As this research shows, moderate exercise will keep your heart and your body in top shape.

Tip 89 Don't Forget to Stretch: But Warm Up First

Stretching exercises can improve the flexibility of the joints, muscles, and tendons, thus making the body less prone to injury. Stretching also increases the flow of blood to the stretched muscle and helps to promote bone growth where there is a stretching motion against gravity. Stretching before your workout tunes and tones your muscles and ligaments before your exercise. Stretching also has the advantage of preventing muscle and ligament injuries when you walk or work out. There is also increasing evidence that stretching has a calming effect on the central nervous system by transmitting relaxing signals along chemical neurotransmitter pathways from the peripheral nervous system to the brain.

New research suggests that you should actually warm up your muscles prior to stretching exercises. This can be accomplished by a gentle five-minute walk or five minutes on a stationary bike or treadmill at a very slow speed. So, in effect, you are first warming up your muscles before you stretch, and then stretching in turn further warms up your muscles, ligaments, and joints before you begin to exercise more vigorously. Think of it as a "double warm-up."

Proper Stretching Technique and Sample Stretches

Stretching should be done slowly, and stretching one muscle group at a time is preferable.

Arm Stretches

Stretch both arms in front of you and hold that position for five to ten seconds, and then let your arms down slowly and relax them for an additional five to ten seconds. Next extend both arms out to your sides, hold for five to ten seconds, and then slowly let them down and relax them for five to ten seconds. Repeat this motion with your arms above your head, and then with your hands clasped in back of your head with your elbows bent as if you are stretching when you get out of bed.

During each of these exercises, gently stretch the arms by pulling or pushing them away from the body and then pulling them back toward the body. Remember to do it gently; if it hurts, you're stretching your muscles too much.

Neck Stretches

To stretch your neck muscles, first look up and hold your head in that position for ten seconds, then relax, returning to a normal head position for ten seconds. Repeat the procedure looking to the left, and then to the right. Also repeat looking down, with your chin resting on your chest for ten seconds, and then return to the normal position for ten seconds.

Leg Stretches

The best way to stretch your leg muscles and ligaments is to sit in a chair and stretch one leg at a time in front of you for ten seconds, then relax the muscles, and then bend your knee and hold that position for an additional ten seconds, then relax the muscles and place your foot back on the floor. Repeat the same procedure with the other leg. You also can accomplish the same thing by pressing your feet into a footrest while sitting on a plane, train, bus, or at your desk.

These simple stretching exercises are designed to develop maximum flexibility of the muscles, ligaments, and joints. Although not as elaborate as yoga or tai chi, they are effective limbering and toning exercises for the body. These stretching steps help prepare the body for mental as well as physical fitness. They help you to get in touch with your body as you contemplate the slow, relaxing stretching steps. Take slow, deep breaths during the stretching exercises for maximum relaxing techniques.

You can develop any stretching routine that feels good to you. Stretching is an individual exercise, and what feels good for one person may not be satisfactory to another person. When you've finished, your muscles should feel relaxed, not taut or tight.

Tip 90 Coordinate Your Meal and Exercise Times

The question always comes up as to when you should exercise. Is it before or after eating? How long before? How long after? Many professional athletes schedule their day's activities around their meals. Also, many fitness enthusiasts become fanatical and inflexible about the time sequence of exercise and meals. Although the average exerciser doesn't have to be as particular about timing walking in relation to mealtime, it's still essential to become familiar, at least in part, with the physiology of digestion.

As food enters your stomach, the heart pumps a significant quantity of blood into the stomach to aid digestion. This does not pose a problem when you are at rest, but if you decide to exercise immediately after eating, there is a conflict of interests. The stomach now has to compete with the exercising muscles for the blood it needs for digestion. If the exercise gets vigorous, digestion is arrested and you begin to feel bloated and develop abdominal cramps. Exercise should, therefore, begin after a meal has passed through the stomach and small intestine. This takes approximately two to three hours after ingesting a large meal, and from sixty to ninety minutes after eating a smaller meal.

Foods high in fat and protein are digested slowly and tend to remain in the digestive tract for a longer time than a meal that is higher in complex carbohydrates (vegetables, fruits, whole-grain cereals, and whole-grain breads and pasta). Foods that are high in refined sugar, like cakes, candy, and pies, can trigger an excess insulin response and should not be eaten immediately before exercise. The excess insulin produced as a result of the high sugar content of food, combined with the exertion of exercise, could drop your blood sugar rapidly. This could result in weakness, muscle cramps, and even fainting.

On the other hand, fasting for long periods prior to exercise is also counterproductive. In order to replenish the stores of liver and muscle glycogen needed for energy, it is necessary to eat several hours before exercising. If you fast, you are depleting these energy stores, and exercise then becomes difficult and tiring without adequate fuel storage reserves for energy.

So what does this all have to do with your exercise schedule? The most important fact to be learned from this discussion on digestive physiology is that it is essential that you don't exercise immediately after eating, especially if you've consumed a relatively large meal. This puts a strain on the cardiovascular system and can even deprive the heart of its own essential blood supply, particularly if you exercise vigorously immediately after eating.

Try Walking an Hour Before and an Hour After Meals

Moderate exercise such as walking, however, forty-five to sixty minutes after a small meal and sixty to ninety minutes after a moderate meal, can actually aid in digestion by nudging the foodstuffs gently along the digestive tract. This in no way competes for the blood in the digestive tract, since the walking muscles do not require every available molecule of oxygen as strenuously exercising muscles do. In fact, the gentle art of walking allows oxygen to be evenly distributed to all of the body's internal organs, including, in this particular case, the digestive tract.

Recent studies indicate a fourfold advantage for dieters who walk before and after meals. First, as we have seen in Tip 85, walking before eating quiets down the appetite control center in the brain and makes us less hungry. Second, walking at any time burns calories directly, as we walk. And third, new studies in exercise physiology have shown that walking anywhere from forty-five to ninety minutes after eating a small to moderate-sized meal will actually burn 10 to 15 percent more calories than walking on an empty stomach. This is explained by what is called the *thermic dynamic action of food*. What this means is that the actual digestion of foodstuffs, combined with the gentle action of walking, results in a slightly higher metabolic rate, thus burning more calories per hour. And fourth, as previously mentioned, research has indicated that you continue to burn calories long after you complete your walking exercise program. These are four great reasons to keep walking for weight loss and weight maintenance.

Tip 91 Antioxidize with Exercise!

Antioxidants are chemicals that help neutralize the potentially dangerous free radicals that result when your body converts oxygen into energy. If free radicals aren't neutralized, they can give rise to a host of problems, including cell damage and a condition called *oxidative stress* that results from an imbalance between the factors that cause oxidation and the factors that inhibit oxidation. Many antioxidant nutrients are found in primary food sources; for example, fresh fruits and vegetables, grains and oils, yeast, and many other food groups. (See Tip 37 for the top twenty antioxidant foods.) Among the many health claims regarding antioxidants in foods and supplements, however, there has been little discussion of the way the body itself can combat damage caused by free radicals.

Living cells have evolved a variety of internal systems that offer protection against oxidative stress. Regular exercise can influence the equilibrium between antioxidation and oxidation, or the oxidative balance. In other words, regular exercise acts as an antioxidant just like any food or dietary supplement, helping the body to rid itself of free radicals.

Physical activity influences oxidative balance, but it does so paradoxically. During acute phases of physical activity such as strenuous exercise, more oxygen is needed to create energy; therefore, more volatile oxygen molecules or free radicals are formed. During this type of strenuous exercise, highly reactive hydroxyl radicals can overwhelm the body's antioxidant systems and cause injury to the cells and tissues. Hence, isolated strenuous exercise produces significant oxidative stress. However, when physical activity is recurrent or moderate (for example, a walking program), exercise–induced oxidative stress decreases over time as the internal antioxidant systems begin to adapt.

This is a very complicated way of stating that regular moderate exercise is beneficial to your health. Regular aerobic exercise, such as walking, improves the oxidative balance in several ways. It regulates enzyme systems that are responsible for cleaning up escaped free radicals and may also decrease resting levels of free radical formation. To put it another way, sedentary people tend to have poor oxidative balance because they undergo oxidative stress even at relatively low levels of physical functioning, whereas fit people tend to have good oxidative balance because their bodies limit oxidative stress during exercise and during daily functioning.

So the next time you eat foods for their antioxidant properties, remember to continue your moderate exercise program to obtain additional antioxidant protection against those nasty free radicals. The result is that you'll look younger and live longer as well as lose weight.

Tip 92 Schedule Your Workouts

We're all busy, overworked, and overscheduled. You have a million things on your to-do list every day. So how can you make sure that exercise is one of them?

Until your exercise program becomes a habit, it is a good idea to schedule your workout into your day. Your exercise program should be planned to meet your individual schedule; however, when you begin exercising, it's a good idea to work out at a specific time every day to ensure regularity and consistency. You will be able to vary your schedule once you have started the program. Lunchtime, for example, is an ideal time to plan a twenty-minute walk, since it combines both calorie burning and calorie reduction—if you have less time for lunch, you'll eat less.

You can choose to work out in the morning, afternoon, or evening depending on what time of day is most convenient for you. You can also change the times that you exercise each day depending on your work schedule or home activities. Here are the pros and cons of exercising at various times of the day according to the fitness experts to help you individualize your workout schedule.

- **Morning.** The main obstacle to getting in a morning workout is the difficulty of getting out of bed. If you choose to work out in the morning, you will want to leave yourself enough time so that you won't be rushed, especially if you have to go to work or have home responsibilities. Since there are usually few disruptions early in the day, people who walk in the morning are more likely to stick with their exercise plans over a long period of time. Plus the sense of accomplishment, having completed your exercise early in the day, gives you a psychological rush for the first part of the day.

- **Afternoon.** Most individuals feel an energy lag between two and three o'clock in the afternoon, which is related to the body's natural circadian rhythm. It may also be partly due to having just eaten lunch. Some exercise physiologists say that walking midday can smooth out that energy lag by increasing the levels of certain hormones that will perk you up for several hours. Remember, however, that it is not a good idea to exercise immediately after lunch or to skip lunch altogether. Walking for twenty minutes and then eating a light lunch will boost your energy level for the rest of the day.
- **Evening.** Due to fluctuations in biological rhythms, you breathe easier in the late afternoon or early evening because your lungs' airways open wider, your muscle strength increases due to a slightly higher body temperature, and your joints and muscles are at their most flexible. This may be a good time to work out, according to some exercise physiologists. However, if you've had an extremely difficult day and you're dead tired, revving yourself up for exercise may seem more like a chore than fun. Also, never exercise near bedtime because the increased energy level that follows the exercise may make it difficult to fall asleep.

Remember the choice is yours. Exercise according to your own biological clock and how you feel, and also according to your own time schedule. It's your body, so listen to it, and it will respond to you with boundless energy and pep when you work out regularly.

Tip 93 Don't Fall for These Exercise Myths

Don't be fooled by these common exercise myths.

Myth: The More You Perspire, the More Calories You Burn

Just because you sweat an extra amount doesn't mean you're burning extra calories. The key to burning more calories and losing more weight is twofold. First of all, it's the intensity of your workout that determines how many calories you burn. If you're breathing hard and your muscles feel sore, then you're burning extra calories. Second, and actually more important, is the duration of your exercise. Moderate, low-intensity exercises, like walking for thirty to forty-five minutes, burn more calories than short-term strenuous exercises, without the muscle aches or the heavy breathing. By increasing the basal metabolic rate for a longer period of time, the body burns calories at a steady rate while exercising and even continues to burn calories, at a lower rate, after the exercise is finished. This is because the basal metabolic rate doesn't slow down immediately after your longer-duration moderate exercise.

Myth: Lifting Heavy Weights Burns More Calories

Lifting heavy weights does burn more calories initially; however, since this activity cannot be continued for a long time, calories are only burned for a short time. Besides, heavy weight lifting can cause muscle and ligament tears and various other tendon injuries. Interestingly enough, studies have shown that lifting heavy weights may contribute to the development of high blood pressure because this is an anaerobic exercise that does not produce oxygenation of all of the body's cells like aerobic exercises do.

Strength-training exercises using light to moderate weights, on the other hand, can be continued for a longer duration, which leads to the steady burning of calories and actually boosts your overall metabolism. This leads to weight loss and the gradual sculpting of muscles for a better, not bigger, figure. Also, these strength-training exercises help prevent osteoporosis, or the thinning of the bones as we age. These exercises also build more muscle, which burns more calories than fat even after you stop exercising.

Myth: A Morning Workout Burns More Calories

The amount of calories you burn has nothing to do with the time of day; it is dependent on the type and duration of exercise you do. Your body can't differentiate between a morning or an evening workout. All your body knows is how many calories you've burned by the duration and the type of exercise you are doing at any particular time of day. It takes burning 3,500 calories to lose one pound of body fat, and the same formula holds true no matter when you exercise. This can take a day, a week, or a month; the calories that are burned are cumulative. In other words, if you burn 350 calories a day walking, you will lose a pound of body fat in ten days (350 calories × 10 days = 3,500 calories burned).

Myth: Running and Strenuous Aerobic Exercises Are the Best Way to Lose Weight

Strenuous exercises burn primarily carbohydrates during the first two-thirds of your workout and then begin to burn fat only during the last one-third of the workout. Walking and moderate exercises, on the other hand, burn fat during the first two-thirds of your workout and then burn carbohydrates in the last third of the workout. You can clearly see that you will burn more calories (fat has 9 calories per gram compared with carbohydrate, which has 4 calories per gram) by moderate exercises like walking.

Strenuous exercises are not only ineffective in a weight-reduction program, but they are dangerous, since they contribute to muscle and ligament injuries, strains and sprains, and have even been known to cause more serious problems like heart attacks and strokes. A recent study from the University of Pittsburgh found that women who rated their exercise as moderate lost a comparable amount of weight, if not more weight, than those women who exercised vigorously. It's the total duration of activity, and not the intensity of activity, that burns more calories. Weight loss occurs more gradually and more effectively in a moderate exercise program like walking. Moderate exercise also contributes to the maintenance of weight loss for as long as you exercise regularly.

Tip 94　Walk the Pounds Away

Walking is a great form of moderate exercise that not only helps you lose weight, but is also healthy for your heart. The great part about walking as an exercise is that you aren't limited to a particular time or location. Walking doesn't require special clothes or equipment. You don't need to join a fancy gym. You can walk before or after work, or if you drive to work, you can park your car a block or two from the office and walk the rest of the way. If you take the bus or train, get off a stop before your station and walk. An enclosed mall could be the perfect place for your walk in bad weather. You can even walk on your lunch break for a refreshing break from the office.

Walking is the ideal aerobic exercise for good health, fitness, and weight loss without the dangers of strenuous exercise. If you want to lose weight permanently, then the energy burned during your exercise should come from fats and not from carbohydrates. During the first twenty to thirty minutes of moderate exercise like walking, only one-third of the energy burned comes from carbohydrates, whereas two-thirds comes from body fats. During short bursts of exercise, two-thirds of the energy burned comes from carbohydrates and only one-third from body fat. It stands to reason, then, that a continuous exercise, like walking, which burns primarily body fat, is a lot better for permanent weight reduction than short spurts of strenuous exercise.

Because strenuous exercise burns carbohydrates it causes a drop in blood sugar, which actually increases your appetite. Walking, on the other hand, redirects blood away from the stomach to the exercising muscles and decreases appetite. Walking also increases the body's metabolic rate, which helps to burn calories at a faster rate.

Walk Off Unwanted Calories and Fat

The only way to beat the battle of the bulge is to burn those unwanted pounds away. Walking burns approximately 350 calories per hour, so you can lose one pound of body fat for every ten hours you walk. A twenty-minute brisk walk daily will burn enough calories to help you lose weight quickly. Ten minutes twice a day is just as good. The following table will give you an idea of the energy expended in walking, which is actually the number of calories burned per minute or per hour, by walking at different speeds.

Walking Speed	Calories Burned per Minute	Calories Burned in Thirty Minutes	Calories Burned in Sixty Minutes
Slow (2 mph)	4–5	130–160	260–320
Brisk (3 mph)	5–6	160–190	320–380
Fast (4 mph)	6–7	190–220	380–440
Race (5 mph)	7–8	220–260	440–520

A pound of body fat contains approximately 3,500 calories. When you eat 3,500 more calories than your body needs, it stores those calories as a pound of body fat. If you reduce your intake by 3,500 calories, you will lose a pound. It doesn't make any difference how long it takes your body to store or burn these 3,500 calories. The result is always the same. You either gain or lose one pound of body fat, depending on how long it takes you to accumulate or burn up 3,500 calories.

You can lose weight by just walking. When you walk at a speed of 3 mph for one hour every day, you will burn up 350 calories each day. Therefore, if you walk one hour a day for ten days, you will burn up a total of 3,500 calories. Since there are 3,500 calories in each pound of fat, when you burn up 3,500 calories by walking you will lose a pound of body fat. You will continue to lose one pound of body fat every time you complete ten hours of walking at a speed of 3 mph. It works every time!

Twenty minutes of walking six days a week is all you need. Walking twenty minutes outdoors or indoors on a treadmill will provide you with maximum cardiovascular fitness, good health, and boundless energy. It will help you burn the extra calories needed to lose weight and also decrease your appetite. This walking plan will also provide the fuel that powers your energy level throughout your day.

When you first start your walking program, pick a level terrain, since hills place too much strain and stress on your legs, hips, and back muscles. Make sure you walk at a brisk pace (approximately 3 to 3.5 mph) for maximum efficiency. When you begin walking, your respiration and heart rate will automatically become faster; however, if you feel short of breath or tired, then you're probably walking too fast. Slow down or stop whenever you are tired or fatigued, and then resume walking after resting.

When you walk, concentrate on maintaining a natural, efficient gait and putting energy into each step. Maintain erect posture while walking, and every so often contract your abdominal muscles to strengthen your abs. Walk with your shoulders relaxed and your arms carried in a relatively low position, with natural motion at the elbow. Don't hold your arms too high when you walk or you may develop muscle spasms and pain in your neck, back, and shoulder muscles.

The muscles and joints of the ankles, knees, and hips provide most of the energy required for walking. When we overstride or understride, we disrupt the natural walking gait. An easy, steady, unbroken stride will produce the rhythm and gait necessary for the effortless act of walking. Also, avoid toeing in or toeing out during the walking gait because this wastes energy. Concentrate on keeping your toes straight, and your stride will be even and rhythmic.

During the act of walking, your arms should swing naturally from the shoulders. Over-swinging the arms purposely during walking will reduce the efficiency of the act of walking and subsequently tire you out early during your walk. Don't concentrate too much on the act of walking during your rhythmic stride, and you will allow the muscles to relax and perform more efficiently. You'll begin to feel relaxed and comfortable as your stride becomes smooth and effortless.

Tip 95 Slow and Steady Wins the Race

Losing weight through a moderate exercise program and healthy diet is a gradual process. The most important point to note is that so long as you stick with the moderate walking program, the chance of regaining back the weight is minimal. This is because the body has gone through a time-consuming metabolic process in which the adjustment to the weight loss and weight maintenance has been gradual. Consequently, no rapid weight gain has been noted in people who have been on a continuous exercise program.

Don't Worry About Distance or Speed

In order to begin an exercise program, you do not have to be an exercise fanatic. You do not have to be a jogger or an aerobic exercise junkie to accrue the benefits of an aerobic walking program. The amount of time you exercise every day is more important than the speed or intensity. If you walk twenty minutes every day, it doesn't make much difference whether you are walking 2.5, 3, 3.5, or 4 miles per hour. You are still burning calories, losing weight, and developing physical fitness. In other words, it doesn't matter how far you walk or how fast you walk, as long as you walk regularly.

This type of walking activity falls into the aerobic form of exercise, in which you are taking in oxygen as fast as you are burning it up. This is an efficient use of energy. Anaerobic exercise, on the other hand, is the opposite condition, which is caused by overexertion, working muscles beyond their capacity—for example running fast or lifting heavy weights. This type of anaerobic exercise leads to the buildup of lactic acid in the muscles, causing pain, discomfort, and fatigue, a condition known as *oxygen debt*.

In order to keep your walk a moderate aerobic exercise, you should walk at a speed between 2.5 and 3.5 miles per hour. If you increase your speed beyond 4 miles per hour, the upper arms and shoulders swing too fast and the lower leg muscles have to work too hard to compensate, thus producing wasteful energy expenditure. It is important that you walk at a comfortable speed, one that does not leave you breathless.

Tip 96 Walk with Weights to Lose More Weight

There is no need to engage in strenuous aerobic exercises or to lift heavy weights at the gym (either free weights or machine weights) to achieve cardiovascular fitness, weight loss, and improved lean muscle mass. When you walk with light one- or two-pound hand-held weights, you build muscle mass, which speeds up your metabolism because muscle tissue burns more calories than fat cells burn. The combination of the fat-burning aerobic walking exercise and the muscle-building exercise of walking with handheld weights enables you to burn fat as you lose weight and develop a new and improved, lean and firm figure.

Power Diet-Step

My Power Diet-Step® plan simply combines the aerobic benefits of walking with the strength-training benefits of lifting light one- or two-pound handheld weights in each hand. When you combine your twenty-minute aerobic walk with this strength-training exercise, you have the advantage of a "double blast" of calorie burning for weight loss while trimming and toning your body.

First of all, your aerobic walking burns approximately 350 calories per hour, or 117 calories every twenty minutes. The strength-training addition of using handheld weights while walking burns another 175 calories per hour, or 58 calories every twenty minutes. Strength-training exercises (walking with weights) increases the body's basal metabolic rate, which in turn burns additional calories. So you burn a total of 175 calories every twenty minutes when you walk with weights and therefore lose more weight, more quickly.

When you walk with handheld weights, walk with a natural arm swing, as you do when you normally walk. Your arms should hang down naturally at your sides. Hold the weights with your palms facing your body. As you walk, alternately swing your arms gently, bending your elbows slightly with each stride. You can also exaggerate this arm swing by holding the weights, palms facing the body, with your elbows bent at approximately 90° angles. Move your arms forward and backward in a pumping motion similar to the arm motion used by runners.

Walkers burn approximately 50 percent more calories doing the Power Diet-Step using handheld weights than by just walking without weights. As an added bonus, walking with weights builds lean muscle mass, which burns an additional 50 calories an hour per pound of muscle. This exercise is ideal in helping to prevent osteoporosis, since walking with handheld weights puts the tension on the bones and muscles that is essential in preventing bone loss. Walking with weights will also help to improve cardiovascular fitness, thus lowering blood pressure and also helping to reduce the incidence of heart disease and stroke.

If you want to add strength training to your regular walking workouts, start by adding two days of walking with weights to your six-day-a-week regimen. (See Tip 97.) If you desire more muscle toning and upper body strengthening exercises, you can increase the walking workout with handheld weights to three times per week.

Tip 97 Give Yourself Six Weeks

It's not always easy to start an aerobic walking program. With a million other things to do every day, it takes motivation to get in the habit of exercising on a regular basis. Set yourself a goal of working out regularly, ideally six days a week, for six weeks. In six weeks' time, you'll notice so many positive changes in your health and your physique that you're bound to be hooked on working out for life!

If you walk for just twenty minutes, six days a week, within six weeks you will begin to notice differences in your appearance, as well as many changes brought about by your improved aerobic fitness:

- The abdominal muscles will be firm and support the internal organs better, giving you a flatter stomach.
- Leg strengthening and loss of fat in the thigh muscles will make your thighs more slender.
- Your gluteus maximus will be toned and shaped, giving you a firmer posterior.
- The improved tone of the triceps and biceps muscles of the upper arm and the fat loss from the upper arm will combine to form a leaner, shapelier arm.
- The pectoral muscles of the chest will lift the breasts and enhance your figure.
- With increased aerobic training, the efficiency of your lungs, heart, and circulation will be improved, adding more energy to your day.
- A regular walking program will improve your sleep without the use of sedatives or tranquilizers.
- Your heart muscle will pump blood more efficiently, which will help to lower your blood pressure and improve your overall cardiovascular fitness.

- As you continue on your walking program your physical fitness and stamina will increase.
- Walking burns calories and increases your metabolic rate, and a consistent walking program will ensure weight loss that stays lost forever.

Tip 98 Don't Let a Rainy Day Slow You Down

Don't wait until the weather is better to go out and walk. There's no excuse for not exercising at home on any day when the weather is too cold or windy or too hot. But be careful about exercising outdoors when it's very hot or humid. Heat exhaustion and, in extreme instances, heat stroke are complications frequently found in those exercise nuts that you see running on hot, humid days. Remember, it's not necessary to walk outdoors if the weather is extremely cold, windy, wet, hot, or humid.

Here are some options to keep in mind when the weather's not ideal for an outdoor walk:

- **Ride a stationary bike.** Pedal at a comfortable rate of 10 to 15 miles per hour for twenty minutes. To avoid fatigue, you can divide those twenty minutes into two ten-minute sessions.
- **Walk on a treadmill.** The treadmill is an effective way to burn calories and build cardiovascular fitness. With a treadmill, you can walk for exercise just as you would outdoors, rain or shine!
- **Swim.** Twenty minutes of swimming provides the same aerobic conditioning and cardiovascular fitness benefits as walking and indoor exercises. Swimming has the added benefit of being easy on the joints, especially if you have any form of arthritis or back problems. If you have access to an indoor or outdoor swimming pool, twenty minutes of swimming will fit the bill perfectly.
- **Try an elliptical fitness machine.** This type of machine combines the movement of a treadmill and a stair-climber.

Your feet loop forward to simulate walking, but the footpads rise and fall with your feet. The elliptical motion provides a no-impact type of exercise, which is great if you have arthritis or knee or back problems that make walking difficult. For maximum exercise, an elliptical machine with dual cross-trainer arms, which move back and forth as you stride, rather than stationary arms, burns more calories and uses more muscle groups.

- **Walk the mall.** If you don't like to exercise at home or at the gym when the weather's bad, an indoor mall can be just the place to take your twenty-minute walk. Many malls open early before the stores open to accommodate mall walkers. If you have access to one of these enclosed malls, then by all means get out there and walk. Remember to put vigor, vim, and pep into your mall walk step and keep your eyes straight ahead, so that you won't be window-shopping instead.

Tip 99 Check Out This Handy Exercise Cheat Sheet

No diet will work if it isn't flexible. Sometimes you can't help but splurge with a diet-unfriendly treat. But just because you cheat a little doesn't mean you have to live with the extra calories. Try walking them off instead! The following table shows how many minutes of walking at a brisk pace of 3 miles per hour are necessary to burn up the caloric value of each snack and treat listed:

Treat	Minutes of Walking	Treat	Minutes of Walking
American cheese (1 slice)	16	Apple (medium)	15
Apple juice (6 ounces)	17	Bagel (1)	23
Banana (medium)	16	Beer (12 ounces)	30
Bologna sandwich	50	Candy bar (1 ounce)	45
Cake (1 slice pound cake)	63	Chocolate bar with nuts	28
Cheese crackers (6)	35	(1 ounce)	
Chicken, fried (3 pieces)	50	Cheese steak (½)	55
Corn chips (small pack)	33	Chocolate cookies (3)	25
Frankfurter and roll	50	Doughnut (jelly)	40
Hamburger (4 ounces)	73	French fries (3 ounces)	50
and roll		Ice cream cone	30
Ice cream sundae	75	Milk shake, chocolate	42
Muffin, blueberry (small)	25	(8 ounces)	
Peanut butter crackers (6)	50	Orange juice (6 ounces)	16
Pie, apple (1 slice)	46	Peanuts, in shell	37
Potato chips (small pack)	33	(2 ounces)	
Pretzels (1 soft)	30	Pizza (1 slice)	40

Treat	Minutes of Walking	Treat	Minutes of Walking
Pretzels, hard (3 small)	30	Shrimp, cocktail (6 small)	18
Soda, regular (12 ounces)	24	Tuna on whole wheat	41
Whiskey, rye (1 ounce)	17	(2 ounces)	
Wine, Chablis (4 ounces)	14		

If your favorite snack food is not listed in the table, you can easily figure out the time you have to walk to burn it off. Walking at a brisk pace (3 miles per hour) burns approximately 6 calories per minute, so to calculate how many minutes you need to walk to burn off your snack, just take the calorie count and divide it by 6.

Tip 100 Remember: It's Easier to Get in Shape than Out of Shape

There's no need to get discouraged if you miss a couple of days of your exercise program or panic if you don't hit the gym for a week or two straight. Many people don't start an exercise program because they are worried they won't be able to keep it up regularly. But instead of focusing on the negative and worrying about whether or not you'll be able to keep up with the program, it's important to keep in mind that it's easier to get in shape than out of shape.

The body is remarkable and tends to hold onto its fitness gains long after you've stopped exercising. Even if you miss a few days or a week of exercise, or even a few weeks in a month, there is no need to worry. Once you have been conditioned physically, it takes a lot longer to get out of shape than it took you to get into shape. The rate of regression depends on how long you've been exercising and how fit you are. Most people lose muscle strength at about one-half the rate at which they gained it. So if you've been exercising regularly for three months and have to discontinue for any reason, it could take up to six months for your body to fall back to its pre-training state.

If you've been walking for approximately two or three months, your aerobic capacity starts to decrease in the first two to three weeks after you've stopped exercising, but it can take almost four to six months before fit exercisers get back to the prefitness level where they started. Aerobic exercising decreases the bad LDL cholesterol and increases the good HDL cholesterol after you've been on your exercise program for approximately two to three months. Studies show that it took at least three months for those cholesterol levels to return to their original pre-exercise levels after the exercise was discontinued. When exercisers resumed their program, it took them only half the time to return to their original levels of fitness.

So don't panic if you have to take a short break from your exercise program. The benefits that you've worked so hard for are long-lasting, and they can be obtained again in half the time. It's motivating to think how far each workout takes you toward getting trim and fit, and staying fit for longer.

Afterword

Enjoy Life and Live Longer

By following these 100 tips to lose weight and keep it off for good, you will not only look great, but you'll be doing your body and health a favor as well.

Studies show that excess weight causes cardiovascular disease with a significant increase in mortality and that life expectancy improves following weight reduction. Overweight people have a significantly higher incidence of hypertension than non-overweight persons. The excess body weight demands a higher cardiac output (pumping out blood) to meet the increased metabolism of an overweight body. This, in turn, causes the left ventricle chamber of the heart to gradually enlarge because of this extra workload. The combined effect of obesity, hypertension, and heart enlargement may eventually lead to heart failure. Weight reduction can lower both the systolic and diastolic blood pressures, if it is accomplished before the complications of heart enlargement and heart failure occur.

Excess weight also causes an alteration of the body chemistry and metabolism. The blood-sugar goes up dramatically with obesity, often leading to the development of diabetes. The uric acid in the blood becomes elevated, often leading to kidney stones and attacks of gout. Obese people have higher levels of triglycerides (sugar fats) and the "bad" LDL cholesterol. They also have lower blood levels of the "good" HDL cholesterol. These altered blood fats can eventually lead to severe coronary artery disease. These abnormal blood chemistries can be reversed to normal levels, if weight reduction occurs before permanent complications result.

And if all these risks of being overweight weren't bad enough, here's more evidence that being overweight is dangerous to your health. *Obesity, just by itself, has been listed as an independent risk factor for coronary heart disease.* Newer data from the 26-year follow-up statistics in the *Framingham Heart Study* demonstrated that excess weight, just by itself, was enough to cause a significant increase in the risk of coronary heart disease and premature death in both women and men.

To live a healthier, longer life and to win the war against obesity, you need only to heed these two simple and effective precepts: follow a low-fat, high-fiber, lean protein diet, and engage in a regular aerobic exercise program. These two easy methods of diet and exercise will effectively reduce your weight permanently, lower your blood fats and help to reduce your risk of hypertension, heart disease, strokes and certain forms of cancer. In short, these steps will add years to your life and life to your years.

Index